Flat Belly Diet!

A BREAKTHROUGH PLAN
FROM THE EDITORS OF **Prevention**®

Flat Belly Diet!

LOSE up to 15 LBS in 32 days!

A FLAT BELLY IS ABOUT FOOD & ATTITUDE.
PERIOD. (NOT A SINGLE CRUNCH REQUIRED)

BY LIZ VACCARIELLO, Editor-in-Chief, with Cynthia Sass, MPH, RD

RODALE®

Back cover photographs (bottom left) by Kristine Larsen; (top right) by Marcus Nilsson, food styling by Anne Disrude, prop styling by Deborah Williams for Pat Bates and Associates; (tape measure photo) by Ted Morrison

Cover design by Jill Armus

Illustrations © Eric Feng
Interior exercise photos © Tom MacDonald/Rodale Images
Before/after/now photos by Kristine Larsen

Library of Congress Cataloging-in-Publication Data

Flat belly diet! : a flat belly is about food & attitude, period (not a single crunch required) / Liz Vaccariello, editor-in-chief ; with Cynthia Sass.
    p.   cm.
Includes index.
ISBN-13 978–1–59486–850–4 hardcover
ISBN-10 1–59486–850–6 hardcover
1. Reducing diets. 2. Abdomen. I. Vaccariello, Liz. II. Sass, Cynthia.
RM222.2.F535 2008
613.2'5—dc22   2007048944

2 4 6 8 10 9 7 5 3 1 hardcover

RODALE
LIVE YOUR WHOLE LIFE™

We inspire and enable people to improve their lives and the world around them

For more of our products visit **rodalestore.com** or call 800-848-4735

For the millions who bemoan their bellies,
so they can learn to love them instead.

—Liz and Cynthia

Contents

Acknowledgments

We dedicate *The Flat Belly Diet* to the readers of *Prevention*—all 11 million of you—who have told us in no uncertain terms that belly fat is your biggest physical challenge.

Our gratitude to the Rodale family. For generations, through their magazines, books, and online properties, they have been dedicated to a special mission, that of giving people the tools and inspiration to live their whole lives. Our most heartfelt thanks to Rodale CEO Steve Murphy, whose leadership means Rodale is the kind of company where creativity is nurtured and the highest standards are set—and met—daily. It all starts with the edit, Steve!

Like magazines, books are a collaborative effort, and this one is no exception. Very special thanks to Gregg Michaelson ("Let's make it happen!"), Janine Slaughter, Liz Perl Erichsen, and Jim Berra (the unsung hero behind all things *Prevention*). To Robin Shallow, who never met an idea she didn't improve, and Karen Mazzotta, who is tireless in her enthusiasm and support. And to Fotoulla Euripidou, for her understanding of the *Prevention* audience and for helping us determine whether *Prevention* readers would be interested in this kind of diet book—by asking them!

We'd also like to extend our gratitude to the original members of our initial test panel, which was conducted in summer of 2007. They first opened our eyes to how special the Flat Belly Diet really was. Thank you Mary Aquilar, Syndi Becker, Katherine Brechner, Donna Christiano, Evelyn Gomer, Diane Kastareck, Patty Lloyd, Kevin Martin, Nichole Michl, Colleen O'Neill-Groves, Julie Plavsic, and Mary Anne Speshok for devoting your summer to this project and providing us with the essential insights that helped us develop this book beyond daily meal plans. Thank you also Gina Allchin, President–Health Trek P.T.T., who measured each and every one of our panelists with precision and compassion—a tough combination!

You literally would not be holding this book in your hands without executive editor Nancy Hancock ("good to great!"). All thanks to her dedicated team, including Chris Krogermeier, Marina Padakis, Anthony Serge, JoAnn Brader, Keith Biery, Hope Clarke, and Ana Palmiero. And of course, to Ina Yaloff—one of the fastest, most creative writers we've ever known—we offer a round of applause.

Big hugs to *Prevention*'s brilliant creative director, Jill Armus, whose ability to communicate elegance, authority, and strength through color and design have infused the entire *Prevention* brand of products (most recently this book cover) with new vitality. And to *Prevention* fitness director Michele Stanten, whose contribution to and extensive review of Chapter 9 have helped make it one of the most authoritative sources of information on banishing belly fat with exercise.

Thanks also to Miriam Backes, Merritt Watts, Amy Gorin, Katie Kackenmeister, and Kristen Watson, who assisted with coordinating the test panel and fact-checking the manuscript, even during precious nights and weekends. To Lori Conte, Courtenay Smith, and Polly Chevalier: for keeping the trains running on time. And to the smartest photo and art team in the business, including *Prevention*'s Helen Cannavale, Kim Latza, Faith Enmark, Jessica Sokol, and Donna Agajanian. And of course to Rosalie Rung, who helped capture the enormous success of our test panelists on film and video.

Our deepest gratitude we save for brand editor Leah McLaughlin, a colleague and friend to both of us for more than six years. From helping develop the initial idea to making sure the most engaging, authoritative manuscript shipped to the printer and every moment in between, Leah was critical to the launch of this book—not to mention the companion online subscription service, flatbellydiet.com.

Finally, we'd like to thank our husbands, Steve Vaccariello and Jack Bremen, and families (especially Olivia and Sophia Vaccariello and Diane Salvagno!) for putting up with all the late—late!—nights and never-ending conversations about Flat Belly Diet this and Flat Belly Diet that. (Yes, now we can take a weekend off, guys!)

Get Ready for a Flat Belly

It doesn't matter what your personal stumbling blocks are: baby weight, killer cravings, or (say it with me) "getting older." Belly fat is *not* your destiny. I am delighted to tell you that you can, and will, get rid of it. *Prevention* has found a way to target belly fat that is healthy, real, long-lasting, and works for everyone.

Before we get started, I think it's important to do a "gut check." Chances are, if you've plunked down cold, hard cash for a book called *Flat Belly Diet*, you may wish you had someone else's belly, or wish you had your own belly—from 20 years ago.

I want to ask you to change your thinking. Be kind to your belly. No matter how flat or round, jiggly or rock-hard—it's yours, and it's powerful. It's probably the center of some of your most profound memories. Think about it . . . the laughter you've shared, the romantic dinners you've had, the butterflies you've felt, the children you may have carried. All these set up house in—yes—your belly. And for that, it deserves your respect. Your appreciation. And more than a little love and kindness . . . even when you're struggling to button your jeans.

How do I feel about my belly?

I consider it my core strength, and I love to feel it move, twist, support me as I go through life's business. It's where food (one of life's greatest pleasures, yes?) touches down, and there are few things as peaceful for me as that not-stuffed-not-hungry-but-just-full feeling. It's also my meditative center, and I sense the calm overtaking me when I fill my middle with deep breaths. Then, of course, there's the role it played in my pregnancy with twins. Anything willing to expand to host two precious, growing, kicking girls earns a special place in my heart for all time.

But the belly betrays. If I'm puffy the morning after a sushi dinner, that's where my outfit feels tight. If PMS strikes, my belly moans and groans. When I gain five pounds, that's where it shows. And, of course, when I go to take those five pounds off, that's where they stay.

One of the best things about being editor-in-chief of *Prevention* is hearing from all of you and learning—clearly and quickly—that I am not alone in my love/hate affair with this fascinating, troublesome part of the body. Many of you have told me that when look at yourself in the mirror, you overlook your familiar, beautiful features, the favorite nuances of your physique. Instead, your eye travels directly to the areas where your fat resides. And for most of us, that's the belly.

For countless reasons that I will outline throughout this book, the belly starts letting us down around age 40. Sometime between our 35th and 55th birthdays (some earlier, some later and some, God willing, never) the belly pooches, puffs, and starts spilling over our waistbands. First we suck it in, yet it refuses to achieve its formerly flat shape. Then we crunch until our necks scream, while the fat over the sculpted abs muscles remains. And eventually we diet, then watch with frustration as the weight disappears from our breasts and our faces and the belly fat stays put. Eventually, belly fat starts to feel like our destiny—something that even hours on the treadmill or the strictest diet in the world won't budge. . . .

Until now.

Here's another great thing about heading up a brand like *Prevention*. I have deep relationships with the best experts in every area of health, fitness, and nutrition, and it's my job to look for solutions to the health challenges that my readers struggle with most. (Bonus—that help me too!) And that's exactly what I've done.

My quest to find the absolute best way to blast belly fat started when I hired *Prevention*'s new nutrition director, Cynthia Sass, MPH, RD. Her first challenge was to comb the latest research, combine it with her vast clinical experience, and develop a diet that would target abdominal fat specifically. I made a good decision—Cynthia is not only a phenomenal magazine editor, but she is also a registered dietitian with two graduate degrees and 15 years of experience, including countless hours of working with women over 40. And here's the best part: She is passionate about food! I knew that any diet I asked her to construct would be satisfying and delicious, that it would be a way of eating that women could embrace for a lifetime. And boy, was I right.

She has developed a belly-reduction eating plan that is grounded in the latest and most credible science (that you won't find anywhere else!)—and offers the most filling, satisfying, and delicious way of eating that you will ever come across.

But my vision for this Flat Belly Diet went beyond food. I know that any successful diet acknowledges that we eat for emotional reasons as well as physical ones. Not only does the Flat Belly Diet deliver a healthy, satisfying way of eating—one that will rid your body of fat in the place you told us you want to slim down most—but it will teach you how to *want* to eat this way forever. The mental tricks, tips, and strategies are culled from the latest research and are designed to inspire you, motivate you, and set you up for a better relationship with food for the rest of your life!

Belly Fat Defined

When I toss around the words "belly fat," I'm actually talking about two different types: *subcutaneous* and *visceral*. **Subcutaneous fat** is best, though perhaps not most scientifically, defined as the fat that you can see, the "inch you can pinch." Subcutaneous means "beneath" (*sub*) "the skin" (*cutaneous*), and it's no big secret that this fat resides all over. In some spots—your thighs, underarms, *tummy, anyone?*—it may be thicker than in others, but for the most part it's everywhere, even on the soles of your feet. A moderate amount of subcutaneous fat is essential for life—for one thing, it keeps you from freezing to death in the winter. But too much of it causes dissatisfaction with how we look (which studies show leads to even more dangerous health behaviors). And worse: Excessive amounts of subcutaneous fat function as a visible sign of being overweight or obese, which studies show raises your risk for many diseases. But I have some great news: Subcutaneous fat responds immediately to this diet plan.

Before you happily skip pages and move to the diet, let's talk about the second type of fat—visceral—which is much more dangerous and difficult to lose. **Visceral fat** resides deep within your torso and is sometimes referred to as "hidden" belly fat. I prefer the term "deadly." Because of its proximity to your heart and liver, excess visceral fat can increase your risk of all sorts of diseases, from heart disease and diabetes to cancer and Alzheimer's disease. And the most frustrating part? You can cut calories and exercise religiously and still be left with too much of it.

In fact, the only way to minimize both visceral and subcutaneous fat simultaneously is to eat the right . . . fat.

The New Belly-Flattening Nutrient

At *Prevention*, we've been talking about the healthfulness of monounsaturated fat—the kind found in olive oil, nuts, and avocados—for decades. Nearly every issue contains some tip or strategy for getting more in your diet. In fact, we're on such intimate terms with monounsaturated fatty acids that we have a nickname for them—MUFAs (pronounced MOO-fahs). But it wasn't until the spring of 2007 that we realized just how amazing these fats are. That was when Spanish researchers published a study in the journal *Diabetes Care* showing that eating a diet rich in MUFAs *can actually help prevent weight gain in your belly.*[1]

The researchers looked at the effect of three different diets—one high in saturated fat, another high in carbohydrates, and a third rich in MUFAs—on a group of patients with "abdominal fat distribution" or, in language the rest of us non-scientists can understand, belly fat. All three diets contained the same number of calories, but only the MUFA diet was found to reduce the accumulation of belly fat and, more specifically, visceral belly fat.

Bear in mind: *No other nutrient can do this*. And that's what makes *Flat Belly Diet* unlike any other diet book you've ever read. It's the only diet to give MUFAs center stage, to make them an essential part of every single meal. And that means it's the only diet that helps you lose fat in the belly *specifically*! In Chapter 5, you'll read more about MUFAs and their various health benefits, but until then, let's take a broader look at this truly groundbreaking diet plan.

The Flat Belly Diet Program

The Flat Belly Diet is made up of two parts—a *Four-Day Anti-Bloat Jumpstart* and a *Four-Week Eating Plan.* The whole thing together takes just 32 days, which studies show is just enough time to make any dietary change a lifestyle. Then, after you've mastered the program and seen the desired changes in your weight and measurements, I give you the tools to keep your belly flat for life. Even though you may be tempted to follow one part without the other, I want you to start with the Anti-Bloat Jumpstart, then move straight into the four-week eating plan. Here's why:

The Four-Day Anti-Bloat Jumpstart isn't just about beating bloat; it's also extremely important in sparking your emotional commitment to the entire program. The four-day plan includes a prescribed list of foods and drinks you can eat that will help flush out fluid, reduce water retention, and relieve digestive issues like gas and constipation, which can make your belly puff unnecessarily. You'll drink Cynthia's signature Sassy Water and eat healthy foods like fruits, vegetables, and whole grains. When we tested this diet on our group of volunteers, one of the participants lost an amazing *7 pounds and 5 inches in the first 4 days (that's just 96 hours).*

Losing the bloat isn't just a way to fit into your favorite dress again. It's about feeling confident, powerful, and proud of your body. Dropping even a few pounds of unnecessary water weight can be thrilling and can give you a major confidence boost—essential for success on any diet plan. Plus, I've added a second element to the four-day plan: a Mind Trick at every meal. These quick and easy healthy-eating triggers will serve as mealtime reminders that you have embarked on a new way of life—a new way of living with and caring for your body.

The Four-Week Eating Plan begins the morning after you complete the Anti-Bloat Jumpstart, and it's the centerpiece of this book. Every day you'll enjoy three super-satisfying 400-calorie meals and one 400-calorie Snack Pack. Each meal and snack contains just the right amount of MUFA to make that belly fat disappear. How simple is that? No calorie counting. No math! We chose the quantity of 1,600 calories per day because that's the precise amount for a woman over 40 of average height, frame, size, and activity level to get down to her ideal body weight, while maintaining a high energy level, healthy immune system, and strong muscles. It also ensures you won't feel tired, cranky, irritable, moody, or hungry.

But because no plan fits all, we've provided two different versions: The first one's perfect for people who have little time to spend in the kitchen. In Chapter 6, you'll find 84 different 400-calorie, MUFA-packed Quick-Fix Meals and 28 different 400-calorie Snack Pack options. Choose three meals and one Snack Pack a day and you're done. In a month, you'll have a flatter belly and I'll have done my job.

Sometimes, however, you'll want a more involved home-cooked meal, whether it's family night, or the weekend, or you're just a good cook who likes to flex her culinary muscles now and then. In Chapter 7, you'll find more than 80 recipes that all provide the requisite number of calories and MUFAs per serving, so they can be swapped in for any of your required three meals a day.

WHAT ABOUT EXERCISE?

I exercise every day, walking 50 minutes as part of my commute. (I also strength-train every weekend and try to fit in a weekly Pilates class or yoga session, too.) And I encourage every *Prevention* reader to make exercise a part of their healthy lifestyle.

To that end, I asked *Prevention*'s fitness director, Michele Stanten, to devise the exercise program in Chapter 9 for you to follow as you embark on the Flat Belly Diet. Adding a fitness program to the eating plan and mental strategies will mean faster results (it certainly did for some of our testers). And of course, whether you're trying to lose weight or simply maintain good health, fitness is integral.

But what makes the Flat Belly Diet truly special is that *you don't need to exercise to reap the benefits*. If you do exercise, you will most certainly see results faster, and you will gain secondary benefits like improved cardiovascular health and stronger, more toned muscles. But you can still expect to shrink your belly—and lose both subcutaneous and visceral fat—by simply following the eating plan.

If you do not already exercise regularly, you don't have to start doing so right away. I have always been a big believer in the phrase "Small changes, big results." To me, it's more important that you do *something* to reduce your belly fat than it is to do *everything*, only to find that too many changes are too overwhelming to maintain. If you do not already have a workout routine, incorporating a new way of eating into your lifestyle may be change enough for the first 32 days.

Like the four-day jumpstart, the four-week plan isn't only about what you eat. It's about how you think. In Chapter 8, you'll be asked to keep a daily journal—a key predictor of success on any diet. Every day, you'll be prompted to reflect on a particular aspect of your relationship to food, your belly, your body, and your goals. I call these reflections *Core Confidences*—not only because your belly lies at the physical center, or core, of your body, but also because your attitude is at the core of your ability to succeed . . . at anything.

> **Let's review:**
>
> The Flat Belly Diet is:
>
> A Four-Day Anti-Bloat Jumpstart, with
>
> > A daily dose of Sassy Water and
> >
> > A Mind Trick at every meal plus
>
> A Four-Week Eating Plan, comprised of
>
> > Three 400-calorie meals a day of your choice and
> >
> > One 400-calorie Snack Pack of your choice and
> >
> > One daily Core Confidence reflection
> >
> > An *Optional* Exercise Program, plus
> >
> > The foundation for a way of life you can continue for decades.

Throughout this book, look for the boxes titled **Did You Know?** and **Fast Facts** to learn more about fat, weight loss, and general health. These are quick tips, strategies, and bits of information that experts and readers tell me are useful. And don't forget to read the entries titled **Notes from Our Nutritionist**. These are written by Cynthia directly to you, sharing her own thoughts and advice about how to achieve success on this amazing program. You'll also find incredible success stories from the women (and men) who participated in our Flat Belly Diet test panel—and have a flatter belly to prove it!

I hope that by the time you finish reading this book and following this plan, you will have fallen in love with good, healthy food . . . and your belly. If there's one thing I realized when I turned 40, it was that maintaining a healthy mind and body were the absolute most important things I could do for myself—and my family. I wish that for all of us.

The Skinny on Belly Fat

Though disliked and obsessed about by millions of modern American women, body fat is essential. Without it, you couldn't survive. Your cells wouldn't be able to hold together or absorb nutrients from the food you ate. Your organs wouldn't be able to produce the hormones that make you distinctly female. You would freeze to death on a cold day. You'd run the risk of damaging your internal organs just by bumping into a doorknob. And forget ever finding your keys again. Without fat, your brain probably wouldn't even be able to figure out what a key is.

In effect, *you* wouldn't be *you* without fat. Body fat, whether it's found on your thighs, buttocks, or within the intricate coils of your brain, plays a role in nearly every single biological function in your body, and it's impossible to live without it. Of course, there's a fine line between having just the right amount of body fat and having too much.

If my number one dream in writing this book is to make you fall in love with your belly, my second hope is that you fall in love with fat—and by that I mean both the fat in your body (in limited quantities, of course) and ultimately with foods that contain the right fat.

But let's go back to the beginning of the fat storage saga. As our ancestors stumbled across the savannah in search of food more than 20,000 years ago, you can be sure the last thing on their minds was what was and wasn't "fattening." It's a pretty safe bet that the words "Oh, no thank you. I really *shouldn't*" never crossed our foremothers' lips. If they found food, they ate it, because who knew where the next meal was going to come from? Or if it was going to come at all. Their concern was less about making the right food choices than about having sufficient food to keep them going until the next meal. If they were lucky, they had more than enough and stored some of it as body fat—protection against the lean times when there was no food available at all. Packing on the pounds was what our foremothers did naturally. Their bodies—just like ours—were very efficient at storage.

So why weren't *they* fat? Because they were eating whole grains, and a low-salt and high-fiber diet. Vaughn Bryant, PhD, a Texas A&M University anthropologist who studies nutrition, explains that for the past 95 percent of all human existence until now, the most difficult food for humans to find was fat.[1] If you think about it, it just makes sense. There were no Dunkin' Donuts, Domino's pizzas, pints of Ben & Jerry's, or blue cheese dressing. For ages, only wild, roaming animals provided lean, infrequent servings of meat, and the primary fats humans put in their mouths came from nuts and seeds.

They survived, and here we are. We're long past the Stone Age, but our biological programming isn't. It has been thousands of years, and our genes still haven't caught up to our current environment. Instinctively,

HOW FAT CELLS WORK

A fat cell is like a tiny, expandable capsule. So tiny, it can't hold but a microscopic drop of fat. But fat cells prefer not to live alone—they cluster together like little gangs to become fatty tissue. They generally just chill out until they're called into action by precise biochemical signals, usually hormones and enzymes. When hormones and enzymes signal fat cells, they become active, releasing fat into the bloodstream to be used for different purposes.

When you overeat, those extra calories will travel right back into those deflated fat cells and fill them back up. No matter how much weight you lose or how many hours you spend in Spinning class, your fat cells will never disappear. A deflated balloon is still a balloon.

We're all born with the same number of fat cells (about 40 billion, give or take). As we grow up, the number of fat cells we have increases until after our pubescent and adolescent years, when they are pretty much set. In the past, it was assumed that the only difference between overweight people and thin ones was that overweight or obese people had all their fat cells filled to maximum capacity. It's now known that we can—and do, in fact—"grow" more fat cells in adulthood. This is because when fat cells expand to their maximum size, they divide, and increase again the number of fat cells. Some obese people have more fat cells than non-obese people. **But in the end, both the number and the size of the fat cells determine the amount of fat someone has.**

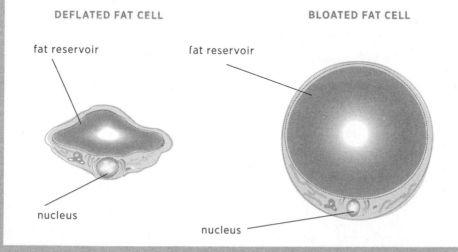

DEFLATED FAT CELL

BLOATED FAT CELL

fat reservoir

fat reservoir

nucleus

nucleus

we're still looking for a backup plan for lean times, so we overeat. Meanwhile, our bodies, not needing all this excess, simply store it. And you know the rest of the story.

The Trouble with Belly Fat

Scientists have known for some time now that excess body fat isn't good for you. Obesity—which, technically speaking, means "overfat"—is considered as deadly as smoking, according to some analyses. For years, obesity was determined by the number on the scale or, just slightly more accurately, by the Body Mass Index (BMI), which roughly calculates your body size while trying to account for bone mass. If your BMI is over 30, you're considered obese—and thus, overfat. (To determine your BMI, see the **Are You Overfat?** box on the next page.)

However, one of the problems with the Body Mass Index is that it doesn't account for your muscle mass. As a result, some athletes—who have a much lower percentage of body fat and higher percentage of muscle—can compute to be overweight or, in some rare cases, obese.

More recently, studies have begun to show that while being obese in general is unhealthy, carrying excess body fat specifically *around your belly* is really, really unhealthy. Studies show that women who have a waistline measuring 35 inches or more are at greater risk for heart disease and diabetes than those whose waistline measurements are smaller. For men, a waistline measurement of 40 or above can be an indicator of the same health risks. Heart disease is the number one killer of American women, and rates of diabetes have reached epidemic levels. The connection between the measurement of your waist and your risk of dying from one of these diseases is no mere coincidence. As you'll learn later in this chapter, belly fat—especially that visceral fat I spoke about in Chapter 1—may actually *cause* these diseases.

Menopause or Man-o-Pause?

If you're overweight or obese, take your pick of things to blame. Alfredo sauce, for one. Not to mention ice cream, and soda, and cake, and cheese, and—well, you get the picture. Eating too much of any food can make you

---

ARE YOU OVERFAT?

When you step on a scale, you're getting a rough indication of how heavy you are, but you can't tell how fat you are. The BMI gets you closer to figuring it out. Here's how to calculate it:

- Multiply your weight in pounds by 703.
- Divide that number by your height in inches.
- Divide that number by your height in inches again.

A woman who weighs 145 pounds and is 67 inches tall (5' 7") has a BMI of 22.7. A woman who weighs 260 pounds and is 67 inches tall has a BMI of 40.7. You can also visit the BMI calculator at prevention.com for an instant calculation.

If your BMI is 25 or higher, you're considered "overweight," but if your BMI is 30 or above, you're "obese." If it's 40 or above, you're "morbidly obese," and your health is at great risk. A BMI below 18.5 is "underweight"—that's also cause for concern, because it indicates too low a percentage of body fat to ensure healthy functioning. An index between 18.5 and 24.9 is just right.

---

fat. Cutting back on cardiovascular exercise is another way to add inches all over, as is skipping a strength training routine. And for some of us, genetics plays a role. But something happens to us after age 40 that makes it easier to put on *belly fat* in particular: Our hormones go haywire.

As estrogen levels decline, your body struggles to maintain its hormonal balance. In the process, body fat—which is extremely important in manufacturing estrogen and other sex hormones, not to mention preserving bone mass—becomes more valuable and thus harder to get rid of. As you enter perimenopause and hit menopause, your body fat distribution starts to look more like a man's, and less like a woman's.

What do I mean by that? Well, you've heard of the term "beer belly"? Male body fat tends to concentrate around the belly area—and it doesn't really have much to do with beer, except for the fact that, because beer is a source of excess calories, it's generally a catalyst for weight gain. Female body fat, on the other hand, tends to concentrate around the hips, thighs, and butt during the years that we're most likely to reproduce. Some

HOW METABOLISM AFFECTS FAT BURN

The word "metabolism" refers to the number of calories you burn per day. Some of that comes from the energy your cells use to perform everyday life-saving functions (like maintaining heart muscle contractions that keep your blood flowing). That's called your basal metabolic rate. You also burn calories through activity, whether that's taking out the garbage or running a 5-K. The last piece of the metabolism puzzle comes from digesting your food, which burns calories. This is called the "thermic effect" of food. The sum of all the calories you burn (basal + activity + digestion) equals your total metabolism, or total metabolic rate.

Being less active affects your metabolism in two ways. It makes the second "plus" in this equation smaller. But you also lose muscle, which reduces the basal number in the equation.

researchers theorize that as estrogen levels decline, the woman's body stops laying down fat in these trouble zones, and starts laying down fat near the belly, like a man's body does.

As I mentioned briefly in the last chapter, visceral belly fat is more dangerous than all-over subcutaneous fat. In fact, it spells real health trouble. According to a study reported in the *New England Journal of Medicine*, people with large hips and small waists produce higher levels of HDL cholesterol, the protective form, than do those with large bellies.[4] (I like to remember the two types of cholesterol in this way: HDL is the "healthy" kind, LDL is the "lousy" kind. See the box on page 21 for more.) Women typically have higher HDL levels—which is linked to fewer heart attacks—than men do. But that all changes when their body fat distribution changes; their risk for heart attack increases. These cholesterol findings are just the tip of the iceberg. Later in this chapter, you'll discover just how deadly visceral belly fat really is.

Not every woman ends up with midsection weight in midlife. Although some women with small waists and large hips can with time develop a midsection large enough that it becomes the broadest part of her body, other women keep the "pear" shape forever. For them, the weight gained in the midsection around menopause is new, but subcutaneous fat is still stored in the hips, thighs, or elsewhere.

Despite what carrying extra weight does to your self-esteem, subcutaneous fat has a necessary role in our bodies. Fat is essential in humans for:

* Energy

* Maintaining proper hormone levels

* Regulating body temperature

* Protecting vital organs

* Fertility

* Bone growth

Subcutaneous fat only becomes a problem when there's too much of it. At that point, it puts a strain on your heart and other organs and, since it is the kind of fat that we can see, it starts to interfere with your body confidence. There's one more notable characteristic of subcutaneous belly fat in particular: As any woman who's been on diet plan after diet plan can tell you, it's hard to lose. But take heart! This diet directly targets that hard-to-lose belly fat. You *are* going to get rid of your belly fat—both subcutaneous and visceral. All you have to do is follow the Flat Belly Diet for the next four days and four weeks and you'll see the results I'm promising and that our test panel of dieters raved about.

Now it's time to look at the other type—the bad boy of belly fat—*visceral fat.*

>>> FAST FACT

From 2 to 5 percent of a man's body weight comes from essential fat, whereas for women, the amount is 10 to 13 percent.

Flat Belly Diet!

V Is for Vicious

Visceral fat gets its name from the term *viscera*, which refers to the internal organs in the abdomen. It lies cloaked deep inside your body where it wraps around your heart, liver, and other nearby major organs. Because it's sequestered beneath a layer of muscle, and it doesn't jiggle when you walk or always show up in your girth—some people call it "hidden fat." In fact, it's possible to be relatively thin and still have too much visceral fat. But this kind of fat can do far more than add inches to your waist: It can subtract years from your life. Carrying excess visceral fat is one of a complex group of symptoms collectively called Metabolic Syndrome, or Syndrome X. The other symptoms are high cholesterol, high blood pressure, and elevated insulin levels. Having just one of these conditions contributes to your risk of serious disease, but your risk grows exponentially as the number of symptoms grows.

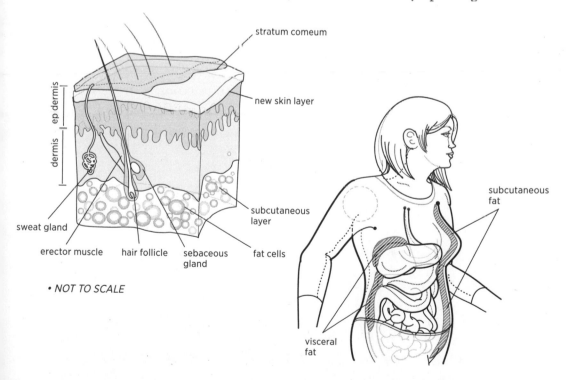

stratum comeum

ep dermis

dermis

new skin layer

sweat gland

erector muscle   hair follicle   sebaceous gland   fat cells

subcutaneous layer

• *NOT TO SCALE*

subcutaneous fat

visceral fat

Visceral fat has been linked to a long list of adverse health conditions, the most serious of which are:

* High blood pressure, stroke, and heart disease

* Diabetes

* Breast cancer

* Dementia

One of the main reasons visceral fat is so deadly is its role in inflammation, a natural immune response that has lately been tied to almost every chronic disease you've ever heard of. Visceral fat secretes precursors to an inflammatory chemical that helps fuel the systemic process that exacerbates early symptoms of disease.

In fact, according to a study published in *Circulation: Journal of the American Heart Association,*[5] visceral fat may have a greater impact on the cardiovascular health of older women than overall obesity. Danish researchers found that women with excessive belly fat had a greater risk of atherosclerosis than those whose fat was stored mostly in their hips, thighs, and buttocks. Here's why:

* The proximity of visceral fat to your liver boosts production of LDL cholesterol—remember, the "lousy" kind—which collects in your arteries and forms plaque, a waxy substance.

* Over time, this waxy plaque becomes inflamed, causing swelling that narrows the arteries, restricting the passage of blood.

* The narrowing passageways increase blood pressure, straining your heart and potentially damaging tiny capillaries.

* The inflammation further increases your risk of blood clots, which can break loose and cause stroke.

But it gets worse. Visceral fat also contributes to insulin resistance, an early precursor to diabetes. Insulin resistance is a condition in which cells do not respond to insulin and the pancreas if forced to increase production to clear the bloodstream of glucose. Over time, insulin resistance can lead to full-blown diabetes, which can severely compromise the entire circulatory system and cause long-term issues with vision, memory, and wound healing.

As if that weren't enough, a Kaiser Permanente study comparing people with different levels of abdominal fat showed that those who had the *most* abdominal fat were 145 percent more likely to develop dementia compared with people with the least amount of abdominal fat.[6] Why? Inflammation again, suggest researchers.

AN LDL/HDL PRIMER

There are several types of cholesterol, but in most cases, the American Heart Association concentrates on two, namely, HDL and LDL. LDL is known as the "bad" cholesterol because it builds up on artery walls and can lead to increased risk for cardiovascular disease and stroke. The American Heart Association considers a level of 130 mg/dL (milligrams per deciliter of blood) or less optimal for most people. HDL is the healthy cholesterol. It transports LDL cholesterol out of the bloodstream and deposits it in the liver, where it can be processed and excreted. High amounts of HDL (60 mg/dL or higher) gives some protection from heart disease.

The ratio of HDL to total cholesterol is a very good way of measuring cardiovascular risk. Most physicians consider a ratio of 4 or under excellent. A person with total cholesterol of 200 mg/dL and an HDL of 50 mg/dL (total/HDL ratio = 4) has a lower risk of heart disease and stroke than someone with a total of 180 mg/dL and an HDL of 30 mg/dL (total/HDL ratio = 6).

Waist Size: The One Number You Need to Remember

I know, all that bad belly fat news was tough to swallow. You're probably racking your brain right now trying to remember your cholesterol levels, your blood glucose levels, your blood pressure, your . . . what are you forgetting? . . . Oh, no! Is that dementia?

Don't panic. All these numbers are important, of course. But the most important number is one you don't need a doctor's appointment to get. It turns out that your waist size, rather than your weight, may be the most critical indicator of your future health.

In research published in the medical journal *Lancet*, doctors concluded that *a person's waist measurement is a more accurate forecaster of heart attacks than the BMI.*[7] The National Institutes of Health (NIH) have set a waist measurement cutoff point at above 35 inches for women and 40 inches for men—*no matter how much you actually weigh*—as an unhealthy sign of excess visceral fat.[8]

A measurement that specifically reflects the concentration of fat around your belly is the waist-to-hip ratio, as opposed to measuring around your hips or thighs. In other words, it's just slightly more targeted to belly fat. Analyzing data from 27,000 people in 52 countries, scientists found that heart attack sufferers had similar BMIs, but higher waist-to-hip ratios,

Did You Know (?)

According to the Centers for Disease Control and Prevention, more women die from heart disease alone than from every type of cancer *combined*.

than those who'd never had a heart attack. Which number would you rather track?

The waist-to-hip ratio compares the measurement of the narrowest part of your waist to the broadest section of your hips. Your waist measurement should be taken in the spot that falls between the rib cage and the hip bone as viewed from the front.

Your hip measurement is truest if you turn sideways to the mirror and make sure you incorporate your derriere in the measurement. (Sorry, it's true.) Now, divide your waist measurement by your hip measurement. For example, a woman with a 30-inch waist and 37-inch hips has a waist/hip ratio of 0.7.

According to the Centers for Disease Control and Prevention, a healthy waist-to-hip ratio for women should not exceed 0.8.[9]

Other Ways to Measure Visceral Fat

As we understand more about the dangers of visceral fat, researchers are developing increasingly more accurate—and expensive—ways to measure it. The latest test, as we go to press with this book, is one that detects levels of a protein called RBP4 (retinol binding protein 4), which is produced in higher quantities in visceral fat compared with subcutaneous fat. In overweight people, blood levels of RBP4 are double or triple the amount compared with normal-weight people. But other tests are also used, including:

CT (CAT) Scan

A computed tomography (CT) scanner uses radiation to create cross-sectional pictures of the body. The image results in a cross section of your belly that shows very clearly how much fat surrounds your organs. The latest scanners can image a whole body in less than 30 seconds.

MRI

Magnetic resonance imaging (MRI) uses powerful magnets and radio waves to create pictures without the use of radiation. Images generated by

>>> FAST FACT

A recent Mayo Clinic study found that even a modest gain in visceral fat causes dysfunction of blood vessel linings. Even more surprising: The study participants were all lean and healthy. So you don't have to be "fat" to have an enemy in visceral fat.[10]

MRI are generally superior to CT scans because they are more finely detailed. They are also generally more expensive than CT scans.

DXA

Dual-energy X-ray absorptiometry (DXA) uses less radiation than a CT scan to assess visceral fat, and is less expensive. It's typically used to assess bone mineral density, but can also be a valuable tool in assessing body composition.

Sonogram/Ultrasound

Ultrasound machines send out high-frequency sound waves that reflect off body structures of different densities to create a picture called a sonogram. As with MRI, there is no radiation exposure with this test. A clear, water-based conducting gel is applied to the skin over the area being examined to improve the transmission of the sound waves. The ultrasound transducer (a handheld probe) is then moved over the abdomen to produce an image of what's inside.

Bioelectrical Impedance Analysis

Bioelectrical impedance analysis (BIA) is portable, easy to use, and low-cost compared to the procedures described above. A BIA involves circulating a very faint electrical current through the body. A device then calculates the resistance the current encounters as it travels through the body, and computes body fat percentage based on height, weight, and speed of the current. A faster current translates to a lower body fat percentage because electricity travels faster through muscle (a greater percentage of water is found in muscle) than it does through fat.

Beyond Your Belly

Remember, by using an inexpensive tape measure, you can most easily determine if your belly is endangering your health. But even if your belly measurement doesn't indicate a health risk, other things may motivate you to lose weight. Any reason is valid. No matter how or why your belly fat developed, you are clearly eager to get rid of it—and to keep it off! That commitment will be integral to your success. Before we get to the eating plan, I want you to understand the one factor that will be key to making your dream of a flat belly come true—and that's your state of mind. Your emotions, stress level, and body image all play a role in how and when you eat—and even how and where you put on weight. That's right—your emotional state can actually cause you to store belly fat. In the next chapter, we'll explore this mind-belly connection in depth, and reveal the secret to succeeding on the Flat Belly Diet.

The Mind-Belly Connection

The relationship between mind and body is pretty solid. Understanding how they work together is key to reaching this—or any—weight loss goal. Why? Consider the role your emotions, attitudes, and feelings play in what you eat, how much you eat, and when you eat it.

I clearly recall the day it dawned on me that my relationship to food is profoundly affected by my body image. It was back in the 1980s, and it was all about a mirror. I had just moved into my first apartment and, needing to give myself the once-over and ensure that my skirt wasn't tucked into my pantyhose before heading out each day, I bought a full-length mirror and propped it against a wall.

For the next month, I smiled happily at the longer, leaner image I saw every morning. Wondering if I'd magically dropped five pounds on move-in day, I weighed myself on the scale at the gym. Nope, hadn't lost an ounce. But boy, did I feel thinner! I was so motivated by this state of affairs that over the next couple of weeks, I decided to maintain the healthy momentum. I ran farther, ate smaller portions, skipped desserts, and took fewer dips into the office candy bowl.

Then I finally got around to hanging the mirror properly. That's when I discovered that tilting a mirror against a wall (with the bottom of the glass closer to you than the top) makes your reflection appear longer and leaner. When I hung that sucker flush and turned to see my profile, I came face-to-face with reality. What I saw was hardly "fat"—just slightly less *flat*. Still, it was a major blow to my body confidence. I drove straight to McDonald's and ordered a Big Mac®. True story.

At *Prevention*, we know from nutritional science—and better still, from years of experience talking to women who have tried many diets—that attitude, emotions, thoughts, feelings, and practically everything mind-related all influence the foods you choose to eat and the way you eat them. That's why the Flat Belly Diet is about engaging your mind in this effort as much as your stomach. Our plan is about moving beyond fears and what you think are your limits and finally attaining your health goals. At the core of the Flat Belly Diet is the perfect food plan. But if you want to see results and maintain them for the long term, you have to adjust your mind. Only if your brain is on board will you have success.

Conquer Emotional Eating

Physiologically speaking, your appetite is controlled by biochemical signals that tell your brain that you're hungry and need to eat, or satisfied and can stop. The problem is, we've all learned to override those signals. We eat not only when we're hungry, but also when we're happy or sad, relaxed, or anxious.

To get a handle on emotional eating, you need to understand why you do it. For one thing, many of us have been conditioned to believe that food can bring comfort (who remembers getting a lollipop after a shot at the doctor's?). And it does, at least in the short term. As adults, many of us turn to food to relieve feelings of stress. (I've been known to lean on spoonfuls of peanut butter when faced with writer's block.)

This message that food brings comfort is perpetuated by popular culture. I cringe every time I see a female television character getting over a romantic breakup by burrowing into a pint of ice cream. Yet there's truth there. Snacking is a common response to boredom, anxiety, anger, and, yes, loneliness. For many of us, years of eating to address everything *but* an empty stomach means we have to relearn what actual hunger feels like.

ARE YOU SAD? THEN BE SAD!

The real cure for emotional eating is developing effective coping strategies, not just seeking out distractions. Here's an example: When you're sad and craving ice cream, cleaning out your closet may direct you away from the freezer, but it won't help you exorcise that melancholy feeling. Too often, we fail to take the very important steps of first identifying the emotions we're experiencing, and second, *feeling* them. If you're feeling sad, watch a tearjerker and allow yourself to have a good cry. Or call a close friend who's eager to hear you out in such times. Addressing the emotion rather than avoiding it is the best way to release yourself from the desire to eat.

READ A FLAT BELLY
SUCCESS STORY

Diane Kasparek
Age: 52
Pounds lost: 6.5 in 32 days
All-over inches lost: 6.25

"For me, learning that Prevention *had put out a call for* participants in their new Flat Belly Diet turned out to be both timely and an unexpected blessing in so many ways," says Diane Kasparek. The 52-year-old nurse, who also happens to be a cancer survivor, calls her cancer experience a defining time in her life. As she reached the fifth-year anniversary of her diagnosis, she decided, "It's time to take off the yellow *LiveStrong* bracelet, shelve the *survivor* identity, and get on with my life."

Part of that decision included going on the Flat Belly Diet. "It was just at that time that I heard about the diet," she recalls, "so I decided to give myself a five-year anniversary gift." Her goal was to shore up her health, shed her excess pounds, and return her body to a complete state of balance.

"It was one of the first times in my life I had ever done anything that was *only* for me."

before   after

The first weekend on the diet, Diane sent her husband and son off to the beach, and she stayed at home alone to concentrate on the food plan. "I realized there is a learning curve with it, so I started very methodically, shopping for the food and making the meals and sitting down, by myself, to enjoy them. I decided to start walking every day, too, and it all just took off from there.

"It's interesting," she says. "As you start to deal with your health issues and get better at it, you start treating yourself better. You connect more to yourself in a lot of different ways. Even mentally you're feeling better. Things aren't as overwhelming. Maybe because you have more energy."

She's in thrall of that newfound energy. In the past, she used to come home from work and plop onto the sofa at 4:00 just in time for *Oprah*. "That was it for me—I was done for the evening. I was tired and maybe even a little bit depressed." Things are different now. The food she's eating and the weight loss have energized her. She's out evenings and wanting to do more and more. "It's as if I have gotten back another six hours a day of my life," she says.

"I know it's just a diet, but I feel so good. And I'm so much happier. Cancer takes away some of your control, but now I feel as though I have a handle on a controllable issue. My body is in a really good equilibrium as far as nutrition, and I feel calmer and more relaxed. Like nothing scary is going to jump out of the closet at me."

NOW

Diane lost six and a half pounds on the first 32 days of the Flat Belly Diet, but her muscle mass and her body fat percentage changed. She feels losing slowly is a good thing. "Do I want to lose more? Sure," she says. "But I realized in the big picture, that's just how it is. You don't gain it or lose it overnight. I really feel as though I've got some fabulous new habits that will stay with me. And I'm going to keep going until I lose every pound I set out to lose.

"I refuse to give up. I keep telling myself, if I could successfully battle cancer, I can certainly battle fat."

Are You Really Hungry? Five Ways to Tell

Although we often don't recognize it, the line between emotional eating and *true* hunger is actually quite clear. Researchers from the University of Texas Counseling and Mental Health Center have identified five ways to differentiate between the two:[1]

1. Emotional hunger comes on suddenly, while physical hunger is gradual.

2. Physical hunger is felt below the neck (growling stomach), while emotional hunger is felt above the neck (a craving for ice cream).

3. When only a certain food will meet your need, like pizza or chocolate, your "hunger" is borne of emotion. When your body requires fuel, you're more open to other food options.

4. Emotional hunger wants to be satisfied instantly. Physical hunger can wait.

5. Emotional hunger leaves guilt in its wake. Physical hunger doesn't.

Recognizing these signals can help you distinguish an emotional need for food from a physical one. The next time a craving strikes, try this: Tune out the signals coming from the neck up. Are you physically hungry? Ask yourself what you're feeling emotionally and how you can meet these mental (versus physical) needs.

Address the Stress Factor

Prevention readers know I believe that knowledge is power. At some point in our lives, we've all remarked at how stressed we are. But do we really understand what stress is? Stress is a response to events that upset us in some way; events that throw our lives off kilter and make us feel like we've suddenly lost control. Recognizing the different kinds of stress—and understanding how each affects us—will help you feel more able to take control.

When scientists study stress, they always differentiate between two types: *acute*, or short-term, and *chronic*, or long-term. An example of *chronic* stress could be having a job you dislike but feel you can't "escape" from. An example of a short-term, or *acute*, stress? It might be as ordinary as having to wait in an excruciatingly slow supermarket checkout line when you have ten minutes to pay for your food and get home to relieve the babysitter—or as life-threatening as almost being hit by a car.

Back in the Stone Age, our species' very survival depended on the ability to respond instantly to short-term stresses like being chased by predators. Today, we're still equipped with a hair-trigger mechanism that overrides our rational minds in an emergency or when we feel threatened. We call it the fight-or-flight response, and it's no different if the stressor is a ravenous beast or an impatient boss. Here's how it works.

The Biology of Short-Term Stress

Stress responses begin in the nervous system. The central nervous system (CNS) responds to orders from the conscious mind, while the autonomic nervous system (ANS) functions independently. If you decide, for example, to take a picture of a friend with your cell phone, the CNS puts into play all the actions involved in completing the task, from having the idea to snapping the shutter. Meanwhile, you will continue to breathe (without having to think about it) and your body will continue to go about the business of digesting food, pumping blood, and fending off harmful bacteria. Your ANS governs these functions, operating without a single conscious thought or action on your part.

Within the ANS, there are two branches: the sympathetic nervous system (SNS) and the parasympathetic nervous system (PNS). In a nutshell, the first revs you up, and the second calms you down. Say, for example, you're crossing a busy intersection and see an out-of-control car heading straight for you. You don't consciously order your heart to pump faster and deliver more blood to your muscles so they can react with more force to get you out of the way; you just naturally jump onto the curb. In that mere millisecond, your brain perceives the threat and kicks the SNS into high gear. Here's what happens next:

* The hypothalamus in the brain sends a message to your adrenal glands near your kidneys, which pump out the hormones adrenaline and cortisol (more on this later).

Did You Know

Certain foods can help decrease stress. A British survey that asked participants to track the food/mood connection found that increasing your consumption of water, vegetables, fruits, fish, nuts, and whole grains, and decreasing your intake of sugar, caffeine, and alcohol, had a dramatic stress-reducing impact.[3]

* Adrenaline increases your heartbeat to twice its normal speed, sending extra blood to the brain, as well as to the major muscles in your arms and legs—so you're better able to dodge moving threats.

* Your memory gets sharper.

* Your immune system goes on alert in case it's needed to fight infection from an impending wound.

* Your arteries narrow—so if you're injured, you'll lose less blood.

* Narrowed arteries cause an increase in blood pressure.

* Your pupils dilate and your vision becomes more acute.

* Your digestive system slows down.

* Insulin production ramps up, overriding signals from adrenaline to burn fat, and encourages the body to *store* it in anticipation of future needs.

All this happens to get you safely out of the way of that car barreling toward you—and, once upon a time, to enable our ancestors to dodge that hungry saber-toothed tiger intent on landing its next meal. When the immediate threat is over, so is the short-term stress. That's when the PNS steps in, releasing calming hormones, and your body returns once again to equilibrium.

The High Price of Long-Term Stress

Unlike acute stress, which has a beginning and an end, chronic stress is ongoing. When your marriage hits a rough patch, your child has trouble in school, you finally get that promotion and your workload doubles, your aging parents suddenly need a lot more care—or all of these things happen at once!—that is chronic stress. The problem is, your body still reacts as if these stresses were acute, yet—and here's the important distinction—there's no calming period. The SNS just keeps doing its stuff, keeping you in a state of heightened physiological arousal as if your very life were being threatened, 24/7. And while this worked for our ancestors—who really did need to live every day in the prehistoric equivalent of a level-orange Homeland Security alert—for us, stress with no letup can take a heavy toll.

Scientists have also learned that daily hassles (commuting in heavy traffic, putting up with noisy neighbors) can exacerbate long-term stress. The more your body's stress response system is activated, the more difficult it is to switch off. And that's a major concern, given that anywhere from 60 to 90 percent of illness is stress-related. Here's how the stress/health connection works:

In times of stress, the adrenal glands secrete an abundance of cortisol. Normally, cortisol's role is to *regulate* blood pressure, cardiovascular function, and metabolism. Your body can easily handle the occasional burst of cortisol triggered by an acute or high-stress moment—no problem there. It's when the stress is chronic and a steady stream of cortisol begins to flow into your bloodstream that things start to go bad. Too much cortisol weakens your immune system, puts your heart into overdrive, and raises your blood pressure. A consistently high level of stress hormones adversely affects brain function as well, especially memory. And excessive cortisol can also interfere with "feel-good" neurotransmitters such as dopamine and serotonin, making you more vulnerable to depression.

Cortisol and Belly Fat

Rest assured, I haven't forgotten why you're here. This is a book about belly fat, so let's turn our attention now to cortisol and its affinity for our bellies. Research has shown that cortisol not only stimulates the appetite but specifically induces cravings for sugar and fat—the most easily burned "fuels" (a good thing for our foraging forebears, just plain fattening for us). This helps explain why many of us eat when we're stressed; it also sheds some light on why it's the Ben & Jerry's we reach for rather than a nice crisp apple. But here's the kicker: Cortisol also signals the body to *store* fat centrally, around the organs. That's right. At your belly. It's nature's way of ensuring that resources are readily and easily available for fuel when the body needs it to perform life-preserving exertion or, for that matter, withstand famine. This all makes even more sense when you take

Did You Know

According to a University of Helsinki study of 7,000 adults, those who regularly worked overtime were more likely to have gained weight in the previous year. This may be due to work stress and its role in the production of cortisol, or simply a lack of time to eat healthfully and exercise.[5]

into account the fact that abdominal fat has both a greater blood supply (so cortisol travels there quickly) and more receptors for cortisol.

Manage Your Stress: You *Can* Take Control!

After each of my life's most terrifying moments—piano recital at 9, gymnastic meet at 12, first television appearance at 25—my mother always told me, to my great surprise, that I didn't look the least bit nervous. If she

SIGNS OF CHRONIC STRESS

- Headaches
- Frequent upset stomach, indigestion, gas pain, diarrhea, or appetite changes
- Feeling as though you might cry
- Muscular tension
- Tightness in your chest and a feeling that you can't catch your breath
- Feeling nervous or sad
- Feeling irritable and angry
- Having problems at work or in your normal relationships
- Sleep disturbance: either insomnia or hypersomnia (sleeping too much)
- Apathy (lack of interest, motivation, or energy)
- Mental or physical fatigue
- Frequent illness
- Hives or skin rashes
- Tooth grinding
- Feeling faint or dizzy
- Ringing in the ears
- Disruptions/skips in menstrual cycle; unusually severe PMS or menopausal symptoms

only knew what was happening inside! As I've gotten older, I have learned a few tried-and-true methods for managing the day-to-day pressures of running a magazine, raising my daughters, and tackling hundreds of other projects, like writing this book. My main tactic is to heap lots of gratitude onto the world's greatest husband and New Jersey's best nanny. After that, I shoot for regular exercise, laughing really hard at least once a day, and actually saying the words "I am so lucky to have you" to my husband, Steve, and daughters, Sophia and Olivia, whenever I think them.

For me, these tactics give me focus, perspective, and calm (on most days of the week!). It's easy for me to tell you to reduce stress by "finding a hobby" or "asking your children to do the dishes more often," but how helpful are these suggestions, really? *Prevention*'s 2007 Picture of Health winner writes in her gratitude journal every day. My husband kayaks on the quietest lake he can find. And an editor friend meditates every morning—an idea I love, but an activity I just can't wrap my brain around . . . yet (I'm working on it). But my point is: Since your sources of stress are personal, so should be the ways you counteract their effects.

However, researchers have targeted certain behaviors that will be helpful for most women trying to manage busy lives, deflect anxiety, and find happiness.

Stress vs. You: You Win!

These are my top seven stress-busting strategies, which will not only help you feel calm and live a more relaxing existence, but will prevent stress-induced weight gain in the process. Even doing one thing on this list will help you take control of stress. You don't need to tackle everything at once (who has time to overhaul their life?). Instead, use this list like a tool kit.

GET CALM! SEVEN STRESS-BUSTING STRATEGIES

1. Get more sleep.
2. Get some distance.
3. Get moving. Every day.
4. Get connected.
5. Get positive.
6. Get centered—self-centered.
7. Get it on the calendar.

Make use of the tactics that work with your schedule and personality. Of course, the more tools you put to use, the more you'll benefit.

1. Get more sleep. At the turn of the 20th century, the average American typically slept about nine hours a night. Can you imagine? Nowadays most of us are lucky to get seven. This doesn't just make you tired; it can make you stressed—and fat. Consistently depriving yourself of rest subjects your body to a constant level of elevated stress. Sleep deprivation results in reduced levels of leptin, a protein that regulates body fat and increases ghrelin, which stimulates food intake. So not getting enough sleep causes your body to store fat, slows your metabolism, and makes you want to eat more. Your body must have enough downtime to revitalize and replenish its reserves. This is especially true for anyone on a diet, because if you're in any way sleep deprived, it's that much more difficult to summon the physical energy and mental focus to stick to any diet *or* exercise plan. I urge you: If you do nothing else on this list, put getting a good night's sleep should be at the top of your Flat Belly to-do list.

2. Get some distance. Take note of the things that cause you chronic stress—and when possible, sidestep them. When emotions run high, you may find yourself biting your nails, leaning on your car horn, forgetting important appointments, even yelling at your kids. If you think about what's bothering you—really think about it—you'll most likely find it's not your nails or your children or the traffic that's the problem. It's that you've maxed out what I like to think of as your "stress reserves" and you need to interrupt the stress cycle. When this happens, remove yourself from the scene. Just walk away. Literally. Around the block or just into the next room. If even that is impossible, just close your eyes, count to ten, and breathe deeply. Those few simple moments might give you a chance to process those strong emotions before you become overwhelmed. Physically, you should feel better almost immediately.

3. Get moving. Every day. Studies show that even ten minutes of physical activity will help reduce levels of cortisol in the bloodstream. Exercise changes your body's biochemistry, triggering the brain to produce beta-endorphins, chemicals that calm you down, regulate your stress hormones,

WALK FOR DEEP SLEEP

A little walking goes a long way toward getting a sound night's sleep. When researchers studied more than 700 men and women, they found that those who walked at least six blocks a day at a moderate pace were one-third less likely to have sleeping problems than those who walked shorter distances. Those who walked at a brisker pace were most likely of all to enjoy sound sleep. Other studies show that a regular walking program is as effective at improving sleep as medication. For walking workouts and a full calendar, go to prevention.com/walking.[6]

and make you feel good. So the next time you feel like pulling your hair out or reaching for a fistful of Fritos, head for the door and take a bike ride or even just a quick walk around the block. A little exercise may not solve the problem at hand, but it will certainly help you cope with it.

4. Get connected. Talking with others can defuse your feelings of tension, but studies have shown that even just being in someone's company—without saying a word—helps alleviate stress. It also promotes good health: Research shows that people who maintain personal and community connections have better health than those who don't.

Where Does the Time Go?

GIVE YOURSELF A STRESS REALITY CHECK

A little time management can go a long way to remedy stress. Keep in mind: Time management isn't necessarily about doing more—it's about doing more of the things you *want* to do. Try keeping a time tracker for a day or two to find out where your time is really going. Set up a daily timetable on your computer or in a journal, broken into 15-minute blocks. Track what you do in each block of time from when you wake up to when you go to bed, and evaluate each day. Seeing how you actually spend your time may help you determine how you can make small changes that reduce your stress and improve your ability to fit in healthy meals, physical activity, or just a little downtime.

(An important caveat: Spend time with people who leave you energized, not drained. If there is any question about which is which, ask yourself this question after you've been with the person: Did I have fun, or did I work hard to make sure my *friend* had fun? The answer to both questions can be yes, but if the answer to the first question is no, you need to find someone else to spend time with.)

5. Get positive. Lose the negative self-talk. I'm referring to that little voice in your head, the one that passes judgment on your every move. Whenever you catch yourself thinking thoughts such as, "I'll never get this report done" or "My house is a filthy wreck," stop yourself and redirect your thinking. Instead, replay the thought, but with a positive spin: "I will do my absolute best to meet this deadline" and "I love this house for all its wonderful memories." Forcing these thoughts might feel silly, but I promise you: It will help you feel more in control of your life, and it will build your self-respect and self-confidence. And, as we now know, that is integral to achieving your health and weight-loss goals!

6. Get centered—self-centered. Before you go any further, I want you to grab a pencil and fill in the blanks:

Below, write the names of the most important people in your life.

_____

_____

_____

_____

_____

When you have completed your list, turn to the next page in this book. *Don't turn the page until you have completed this list.*

Okay. Did you put yourself at the top of your own list? Are you even *on* your list? My guess is that if you *did* include yourself, you were dead last. And that's not surprising, because women have always been socialized to put others first. In fact, most women are so *other-directed* that they completely overlook their own happiness and needs. If I asked you about your relationship with your husband, or your parents, or your children, no doubt you could give me specific, detailed, layered answers. But if I asked you to describe how you treat yourself, how different would the answer be?

When you're trying to change a behavior (particularly a health-oriented behavior like eating better and exercising more), it's absolutely essential to learn to put yourself first. After all, what is a diet, if not a contract between you and yourself? You have chosen to read and follow the principles of the Flat Belly Diet. I presume you've done this for the sake of how you look, how you feel, and how your health measures up. And while you've made a commitment to stay on the food plan—it's far more than that. It's a commitment to put yourself at the top of the agenda, to recognize that you are special and you deserve the time, energy, and effort that's equal to everything else in your life.

>>> FAST FACT

Women who choose lots of foods containing large amounts of trans fats may be at a higher risk for coronary heart disease (CHD). A new study by researchers at the Harvard School of Public Health found that women who consume the highest levels of trans fats have three times the risk of developing CHD as those who take in the lowest levels. Previous studies have shown that trans fatty acids increase artery-clogging LDL cholesterol levels and lower good HDL cholesterol levels.[8]

Now I want you to find a nice sheet of clean, crisp note paper and rewrite the list of the most important people in your life. This time put yourself at the top, where you rightfully belong. Post the list someplace you'll see it often, like on your mirror or the refrigerator door. You'll be amazed how much less stressful life is when you remember to always look out for Number One.

7. Get it on the calendar. Now that you have placed yourself at the top of the list, acknowledge that "Me" time is not an indulgence, but an *essential* factor in your health and happiness, not to mention your success on the Flat Belly Diet. "Me" time is yours to take, if you're willing to say, "This is *my* moment, and it takes priority over everything else." How about starting with 15 minutes a day?

I know what you're thinking: *Hey, Liz, I don't have 15 minutes!* You're wrong, and I'm going to prove it to you. On the first four days of this plan, I'm going to ask you to take two to three minutes before every meal to focus on yourself, your ultimate goal, and how much you can achieve when you put your mind to it. I call these little exercises Mind Tricks, because they're simple tasks that help wake up your brain and draw your attention to the act of eating. If you can manage a few minutes before every meal, you've found your 15 minutes over the course of a day.

As you continue past the fourth day on the Flat Belly Diet, I'll discuss the importance of keeping a journal. Every day, I'll give you another, more involved, exercise in reflection—something I call a Core Confidence. These exercises will help focus each day's journal entry and give you a theme to discuss on the page. And guess what? *Each one takes about 15 minutes.* (Don't you love when that happens?)

Armed and Ready: The Big Three Questions

Now you are armed—with knowledge. You understand the scientific underpinnings of both emotional eating and the body's physiological response to stress. And you understand—and can now master—the unique forces at work in the mind-belly connection. You're also equipped with seven useful stress-busting strategies that will help you manage the stress in your life during this journey of healthy eating.

But the final piece of the mental puzzle remains. Ask yourself these questions: Do you want to change your lifestyle? And if so, do you believe, deep down, that you can?

Before we embark on the first part of the Flat Belly Diet—the Four-Day Anti-Bloat Jumpstart—I want you to take a few moments to reflect on these three vital change-related questions:

1. *Who am I doing this for?*

> There is only one acceptable answer to this question, and that is *you.* And only you. You're probably a lot more comfortable doing things for others, whether it's your children, parents, coworkers, boss, or even your friends and neighbors. But how often do you really do something for yourself? Losing weight, if you need to, is

really the ultimate expression of self-caring, more so than booking the occasional massage or regular mani-pedi. Because losing weight can have lasting effects that extend way beyond tomorrow, or your next high school reunion. Losing weight now, especially if you're overweight or obese, can make the difference between feeling tired and feeling energized. It can mean the difference between a retirement you'll enjoy and one plagued by health problems like diabetes or heart disease. As I noted before, the fat in your belly is the most dangerous and deadly. Choosing to cure yourself—especially with a plan like this that promises not just weight loss, but also a whole host of other health benefits—may be the greatest gift you can give yourself.

2. How can I make the next 32 days easier?

Think Flat Belly *feng shui*. I'm not talking about moving your refrigerator into the basement or hanging a mirror over your stove. I'm simply suggesting that you consider all the ways you can make your office and home surroundings more supportive of your new goal. That means divesting the pantry and refrigerator of tempting food, or keeping all the junk food in the second cabinet from the left. As for your office, you may want to clean out your "junk" drawer as you're getting started. (I don't mean paper clips; I mean candy!)

(continued on page 50)

READ A FLAT BELLY
SUCCESS STORY

Kathy Brechner
Age: 53
Pounds lost: 5 in 32 days
All-over inches lost: 6.5

"I really didn't have all that much weight to lose," Kathy Brechner says. "Only five pounds, actually. But believe me, they were the *toughest* five pounds I've ever tried to get off in my life." She credited much of the difficulty in losing this weight to the fact that she's 53 and hovering near menopause. But her current lifestyle wasn't helping, either. "I serve as a volunteer to our local board of education, so I'm often on the run. I'm eating in the car half the time, eating late at night, not exercising enough, running the kids around to their activities in between. Something had to give."

Kathy was concerned that "something" would be her health because, as she points out, she has a family history of heart disease, type 2 diabetes, and high blood pressure. And so, with the image in the back of her mind of the number on the scale slowly creeping up, and knowing that at this point in her life she was facing the same fate as her par-

before

after

ents, she realized it was time to see what new steps she might take to improve on what she was already doing—particularly since what she was doing simply wasn't working.

That was when she learned about the Flat Belly Diet and its focus on good health as well as weight loss. She was already familiar with the benefits of eating MUFAs, and the healthy style of Mediterranean-type foods. But she felt she needed more. She needed structure. "I think that was the initial attraction," she explains. "I just liked the idea of the 32-day principle. I knew I could do anything for 32 days, so why not give it a try?"

Kathy is clearly a family woman, and at first she was a little concerned about how she'd construct the meals so she could eat with her family. "In addition to a child in college," she says, "I'm dealing with a 17-year-old son, an 11-year-old daughter, and a husband who *lives* for chocolate. But it turned out not to be hard at all. For dinner, I'd select recipes that lent themselves to serving—and pleasing—everybody. That was pretty easy to do because there are so many meal ideas to choose from. And my healthy food concerns were covered, because the diet is all about real food. Because it's not processed or packaged stuff, I felt comfortable giving it to my family."

She says the diet completely changed how she and her family view portions. "My husband looked at the menu I had chosen for one of our dinners and he said, '*One-eighth cup of pasta? Who can get by on ⅛ cup of pasta?'* But we not only could—we did. For snacks, I have a flat wicker tray on the counter and I have small dishes of the different nuts sitting there. A measuring spoon is right next to it because it's just too easy to grab handfuls and scarf them down before you know it. The diet has even

NOW

covered the 'quick grab' for nights when I have meetings. I could have a prepared meal and know I was giving something healthy to my family and still sticking to the diet."

Kathy's family loves eating out, and she explains that with a bit of planning, even that hasn't been hard at all. Recently she took her son to tour colleges, and every restaurant they encountered was happy to tweak the menu a bit for her. She would order grilled salmon on a bed of greens instead of potatoes and then put olive oil on the salad. "I ended up with a meal that looked very much like one on the plan. Eating out is very manageable, if you remain vigilant about portion control."

Is she happy with her results? "I'm ecstatic!" she says. "The Flat Belly Diet brought me to the goal I set out to achieve. Five pounds. Gone. For the first time. And as a bonus, my energy level is so much higher that it's been in the past. I'm not getting any more sleep. I haven't been doing any additional exercise. So it has to be what I'm eating." She adds, "I think every woman at or approaching menopause should know this: There's never a better time to start thinking about your health than *right now*. Keeping your weight down and your energy up get harder as you age, so why not be a little ahead of that curve?"

The Mind-Belly Connection

3. Who's on Team Me?

Knowing in advance what or who will weaken your determination to make healthy food choices lets you prepare yourself for those subtle saboteurs the moment they appear on your radar. For example, you're at a dinner party at a friend's house, and when you politely pass on dessert, your hostess says, "Oh, come on. One bite isn't going to kill you!" For you, perhaps, one bite is never just one, and maybe it can set you on a downward spiral of feelings of guilt and failure.

NOTES FROM OUR NUTRITIONIST

"The Mental Tweak That Will Set You Up for Success"

If there's one thing I've learned from my years of nutrition counseling it's this: To make lasting changes, you've got to believe that what you're getting is loads better than what you're giving up. I don't believe in telling people that it's a matter of willpower or to "just do it." Change has to be important to you.

What's really worked for my nutrition clients is doing some self-exploration and coming to a place where the pros of changing truly outweigh the cons—not because they *think* that's where they should be, but because they *believe* it!

I once had a client who told me she'd never understood those people who'd *really* rather have an apple and almonds than a few Oreos. She always thought they were lying, or had an iron will when they'd pass on (free!) goodies at work and eat the healthy foods they'd brought instead. Then, one day, she had an epiphany. It was a Monday afternoon and she was reaching for the candy dish when it hit her. She'd spent the last week eating healthy foods and had been able to join her family on a bike ride. For the first time in a long time, they hadn't gone without her. The satisfaction she got from that bike ride meant more than the momentary satisfaction the chocolate would provide. In that instant, she really did want a crisp apple and not that handful of M&M's. And her choice had nothing to do with willpower.

—Cynthia

Before you begin, consider having a serious heart-to-heart with everyone in your immediate circle. Tell them why you're doing this, why it's so important to you, what you need from them, and how you think it might affect your relationship. You might need to swap your family's Sunday IHOP stop with a healthier breakfast at home, or happy hour with the girls for a cup of tea at a local cafe. When they realize how important this is to you, they'll listen, and we bet some of them will even want to join in.

Questions Anyone?
Liz answers some of your most common and pressing queries.

Q: *You point out that getting enough sleep is integral to success on this plan. I struggle with this issue and do not want to take sleep meds. Do you have any new tricks I can try?*
A: Here are three very effective new ways to sleep deeply:

1. Slip on some socks. The instant warm-up provided by socks widens the blood vessels in your feet and allows your body to transfer heat from its core to the extremities, cooling you slightly. This induces sleep, says Phyllis Zee, PhD, director of sleep disorders at Northwestern University's Feinberg School of Medicine. If you wear an old-fashioned nightcap, you can achieve the same result.[9]

2. Stay on schedule. People who follow regular daily routines, such as bedtimes and wake-up times, work hours, and regular meals, report fewer sleep problems than those with more unpredictable lives, according to a study from the University of Pittsburgh Medical Center. Recurring time cues will synchronize your body rhythms and sleep-wake cycles, explains Lawrence Epstein, MD.[10]

3. Go dark. Although any light signals the brain to wake up, "blue light" from your cell phone and your clock's digital display are the worst offenders. For a sounder sleep, turn your clock around and eliminate lighted devices from the bedroom.

The Four-Day Anti-Bloat Jumpstart

This chapter is a dream come true for any woman who's ever suffered from a bloated belly. A number of factors influence how puffy you feel on any given day, including what you eat and how you take care of yourself. But this plan will address your bloating—whatever its cause—immediately. In just four days, you'll lose several pounds and inches, which will start a cascade of motivation and energy that will immediately set you up for success on the rest of the plan.

I was in my twenties when I first really understood the phenomenon of water retention. I was a magazine editor in Cleveland at the time, and every morning, the staff met at 9 a.m. sharp in a big new conference room on the far side of the floor. I loved that particular conference room. Not because the chairs were comfortable or because we filled it with creative energy. The real reason I loved that conference room was the lighting—it made my new engagement ring sparkle! It was in that room that I noticed that my ring always seemed to fit more snugly on Fridays. And come to think of it, weren't my pants a little tight as well? And where on earth did this belly come from this early in the morning?

Once I noticed the connection between the mysterious poof and a particular day and time, I started paying a little more attention to what I ate and drank the rest of the week. And that was my moment of discovery: Thursday was pizza night. Every week, I'd meet Steve after work for a pie at Mama Santa's in Little Italy. *And I'd salt every slice.*

Yep, engagement ring or not, bloating can really ruin a girl's day, not to mention her confidence. That's why the Flat Belly Diet starts with a Four-Day Anti-Bloat Jumpstart Plan. This phase will start a cascade of confidence because it promises to shrink your belly—a loss of up to $5\frac{3}{4}$ total inches—in just four short days. How do I know? Because we tested the entire Flat Belly Diet—including the Jumpstart—on women just like you, holding weigh-ins on a biweekly basis. You're reading their stories throughout this book, and you can find more by visiting **flatbellydiet.com**. More than half of our test panel lost at least one full inch from their bellies during the Jumpstart period.

There's nothing more satisfying and confidence-boosting when you're starting a new eating plan than being able to see—almost immediately—

Did You Know (?)

Trans fat may cause more weight gain than other fats, particularly in the belly. According to researchers at Wake Forest University School of Medicine, test monkeys gained four times more weight when 8 percent of their calories came from trans fat than others fed on the same number of calories and the same amount of non–trans fats. [1]

your pants getting looser, your cheekbones getting more noticeable, your muscles getting more defined. It inspires commitment and a desire to succeed. And that's what I want for you to get out of this book more than anything else: success. (Well, that and a permanently flat belly, of course!)

The Four-Day Anti-Bloat Jumpstart Plan has been created for the very specific purpose of eliminating gas, heavy solids, and excess fluid so you will quickly feel and look lighter. Bear in mind: This is *not* a wacky—and dangerous—"detox" plan. You'll be eating whole fruits, vegetables, and grains, and fresh, naturally flavored water—wholesome food prepared in simple, delicious ways. In fact, it's what you *won't* be eating and drinking and doing that really makes the Jumpstart so effective. In writing this book, I was surprised to learn that certain common everyday *behaviors* can cause bloating and water retention—and I'm not just talking about salting the occasional pizza slice. I mean surprising things, like chewing gum or drinking carbonated beverages or using hot sauce. And believe it or not, eating with friends or without. The good news is that, unlike hormonal fluctuations, which can also cause variations in your body's fluid balance, most of these behaviors are entirely within your control. To see how, I think it helps to first understand how your digestive system works.

Digestion 101

Your gastrointestinal (GI) tract is about 35 feet long from top to bottom. Read that again: *35 feet long!* That's about seven of you, lying end to end. And it's all coiled up inside your torso (along with most of your major organs and, yes, belly fat). That's why, when your GI tract is irritated or in any way dysfunctional, it greatly impacts how you feel overall. But before we talk about potential problems, let's go over the basics.

(continued on page 58)

READ A FLAT BELLY
SUCCESS STORY

Colleen O'Neill-Groves
Age: 45
Pounds lost: 6 in 32 days
All-over inches lost: 5.5

"I've spent my whole life on one diet or another," laments Colleen O'Neill-Groves. "I really tried them all—A to Z. None with much lasting success. There was always a downside somewhere." She goes on to explain that on all of the diets, when she *did* lose weight, the first place she lost fat was in her face and her breasts, both of which looked okay to begin with. And her belly—which needed the fat loss the *most*—was always the last place to give it up. Another aspect she couldn't get past was that she was always, always hungry. "I would finish lunch and start wondering, *Okay, how soon can I have my snack?"*

The Flat Belly Diet, says the 45-year-old mother of three, is all things great and good. She calls the food amazing, but explains that for the plan to work, you have to rid yourself of your preconceived notions about things like olive oil and nuts. She kept won-

before   *after*

dering how anyone could possibly lose weight on all the scrumptious food. "The bars were overall a pleasant surprise. And the waffles. Pesto sauce. Pizza. Just great stuff. Sure, on these other diets I had unlimited veggies—but after a while, you can't look at another lettuce leaf. And you never got wraps or avocado or pesto sauce."

Colleen says on this diet, you know exactly what you're taking in and the value of what it represents, in terms of it being good for your body. It made her realize how much junk she was eating in a given day, and how many calories she stuffed herself with without even giving it a second thought. "I'm very aware of my body because I exercise so much," she says, "so if there's ever an opportunity out there to take better care of myself, I'm going to take it."

It wasn't all nirvana, though, admits Colleen. She describes the first four days—the anti-bloat diet—as "not that easy," but adds that it was only four days and "in the end, it was definitely a perfect way to jump-start the diet. I figured I could do anything for four days. Now, when I celebrate a bit too much over a weekend, I actually put myself *back* on the four-day diet to make up for it."

In the first four weeks, Colleen lost 6 pounds. "I'm not that big to begin with," she says, "so I was really happy with my results. I lost an inch on each thigh, an inch around each arm, and a few in my belly—while my breast size remained the same—which is exactly what I had hoped for."

NOW

The primary role of your GI tract is to extract essential nutrients like carbohydrates, proteins, fats, vitamins, minerals, and water from the food you eat and the beverages you drink. These nutrients are transported through the walls of the small and large intestines into the bloodstream, where they're then distributed to wherever they're needed. For instance, when you eat a turkey sandwich, your GI tract breaks it down into bits of carbohydrate (the bread and vegetables), protein (the turkey), fat (the mayo), fiber (from the bread), and all sorts of vitamins and minerals. Carbohydrates, protein, and fat get broken down even further into sugars, amino acids, and fatty acids, respectively. The sugars go to fuel brain and muscle activity (not to mention the doings of every cell in your body), the amino acids get used to build muscle and bone, and the fats get stored for future energy needs or get used to manufacture hormones and other essential compounds.

NOTES FROM OUR NUTRITIONIST

"In Defense of the Post-Breakfast Bloat"

One of the things I've heard a million times throughout my career is, "My tummy is flat in the morning and as soon as I eat anything, it sticks out—that's why I don't eat breakfast." Putting any solids into your GI tract will make it expand—it's a simple law of nature. But in the long run, skipping breakfast works against you. Weight control studies have consistently found that eating breakfast is an important factor for losing weight and keeping it off, for many reasons. Nourishing your body in the a.m. spurs your cells to burn more calories over the course of the day. Without breakfast to fuel your morning activities, your brain and muscles must conserve energy (i.e., burn fewer calories) or dip into precious muscle reserves for energy. Eating breakfast also prevents you from rebound overeating later in the day. If you really want to keep your belly flat, choose a low-volume breakfast that will fuel you, but won't take up lots of space or make you feel gassy or bloated. You'll find these in the Four-Day Anti-Bloat Jumpstart menus.

—*Cynthia*

Ultimately, hundreds of biochemical reactions occur and the chemical end products of that turkey sandwich have thousands of uses. But you can see that the ultimate job of your digestive system is to extract as much nutrition as possible out of everything you put in your mouth.

The whole process starts with saliva. Saliva contains digestive enzymes that help break the chemical bonds holding foods together so they can be easily crushed and macerated by your teeth. These enzymes are pretty fast-acting; if you put a cracker or piece of toast on your tongue you'll notice it quickly breaking down, even before you start to chew. Your tongue helps position the food in your mouth and moves it toward the back of your throat toward your esophagus, the 10-inch connector between your mouth and your stomach. It's different from your "windpipe," or trachea, which connects your mouth to your lungs. When you swallow, a little flap called the epiglottis covers the opening of the trachea to guard against choking. (If you've ever had food "go down the wrong way," it's because your epiglottis didn't cover your trachea quickly enough.)

Once in the esophagus, rhythmic automatic muscle contractions help push the food toward your stomach. There, acids further break down your meal, while your stomach muscles churn the whole mixture into what amounts to a nutrient-dense puree, which is then pushed into the 22-foot-long tunnel that is your small intestine. There, with the help of bile, a fat emulsifier produced by your gallbladder, and additional enzymes produced by your pancreas, your meal is absorbed through the walls of your intestine into your bloodstream in the form of individual nutrient building blocks—sugars, fatty acids, and amino acids from carbohydrates, fats, and proteins, respectively. Vitamins and minerals are also fully absorbed during the journey through the small intestine.

You may have noticed that I didn't mention dietary fiber. That's because you don't absorb fiber. Fiber fills you up, but doesn't add to your overall caloric intake. While fiber does contain as many calories as any other form of carbohydrate—about 4 per gram—your body isn't able to use them for energy. Instead, fiber just moves through your body nearly intact. Along the way, it binds to cholesterol, helping to shuttle it out of your system. A few studies have also found that fiber can prevent absorption of other calories you consume—up to 90 per day.

All the nutrients that do enter the bloodstream travel straight to the liver, which filters out wastes and decides where everything usable should go. Anything that isn't absorbed—fiber, waste byproducts—travels down into the large intestine and finally through the colon and rectum. Before it leaves your body, small amounts of water and minerals are absorbed in a last-ditch effort to extract every last drop of importance out of that turkey sandwich.

Now that you're familiar with your GI tract, let's take a closer look at what's going on when you feel like a beach ball has taken up residence there.

Gas, Solids & Liquids: The Balloon Gang

Think of one of those very long, narrow balloons that you find at a child's birthday party, the ones that clowns twist into different shapes. That balloon represents your GI tract. Now picture the balloon filled with water, air, or solid food. Each of these substances expands the balloon, but does so in a different way. The same goes for the substances that cause bloat in your GI tract.

Air: Air entering the intestine—say, for example, from chewing gum, talking, drinking carbonated beverages, or even smoking—doesn't get absorbed by the bloodstream. Instead, it remains trapped until it can be expelled via a belch or flatulence. Until then, it meanders through your GI tract, causing distension and discomfort.

Solid: It's generally just a matter of time before solid food gets broken down and absorbed. But until then, you're feeling like a beached whale.

Liquid: Just like solid foods, liquid eventually gets absorbed, but sometimes, we retain more fluid than our body really needs.

The Four Bad Guys of Bloat

The Four-Day Anti-Bloat Jumpstart Plan has been created for the very specific purpose of eliminating gas, heavy solids, and excess fluid so you will almost instantly feel and look lighter. Before we move on to the nitty-gritty details of the plan—what and when you'll eat—I want to explain four lifestyle factors that can also influence how prone you are to bloating or retaining water.

1. Stress: Everyone deals with stressful situations; they're a part of life. But many women have to deal with chronic stress, whether they're caring for growing children and elderly parents simultaneously or just trying to balance work and family life in an era that doesn't seem to leave much time to focus on either. Stress triggers a complex sequence of hormonal fluctuations that raise blood pressure and divert blood to your extremities, where energy is most needed. This process allows you to run faster or lift more if necessary, but it also causes your digestive system to slow down significantly, which means you absorb nutrients more slowly (and sometimes miss some). Chronic stress has the same effect, but with the added insult of causing you to crave carbohydrates (read: cookies and cake for some, chips or ice cream for others). As a result of the slowdown, your last meal may stick around in your intestine, causing bloat.

In the last chapter, we discussed how making a mind-belly connection can help you succeed on the Flat Belly Diet. The more focused you remain on your goals, the less sidetracked you'll feel by everyday stress.

Did You Know ?

We can survive six weeks without food, but only four days without water. About 60 to 70 percent of the human body is made up of water, and it's required for every single bodily process. According to the Institute of Medicine, women age 19 and over need 2.7 liters of fluid per day (almost a 3-liter bottle of cola) and men need 3.7.

2. Lack of fluid: You've probably heard you need about eight glasses of water a day. Drinking water and even eating "watery" foods like melon, greens, and other fruits and vegetables has enormous health benefits, including warding off fatigue. But perhaps the most important belly benefit of proper hydration is how it helps maintain your body's proper fluid balance and guard against water retention. It also helps prevent constipation, which can cause bloating. Eight glasses is just a guideline; everyone's fluid needs vary according to activity level and body. But eight is a good starting point. All fluids (and water-packed foods) count toward your overall fluid intake, but bear in mind that not all of these fluids are permitted on the Four-Day Anti-Bloat Jumpstart.

3. Lack of sleep: Too little sleep disrupts the intricate workings of your nervous system, which controls the rhythmic contractions of your GI tract and helps keep things humming along. It also affects your overall ability to manage and cope with stress. It's important to get at least seven hours of sleep a night. If you have trouble sleeping, consult a sleep expert or visit the National Sleep Foundation's Web site at sleepfoundation.org. Also see our three new quick and easy sleep tips—all based on research—at the end of this chapter.

4. Air travel: The average plane maintains cabin pressure equal to 5,000 to 8,000 feet above sea level in order to provide a comfortable atmosphere for the passengers. At that altitude, free air in the body cavities tends to expand by around 25 percent.[2] Pressure changes also increase the production of gases in your GI tract. As the pressure in the cabin drops, the air in your intestines expands, causing bloating and discomfort. Cabin pressurization is also responsible for increased water retention because it impacts your body's natural fluid balance. Add in the dehydration caused by recirculated air and those bloat miles add up. Your best defense is to drink as much water as possible before and during your flight, and to try to walk around as often as possible.

NOTES FROM OUR NUTRITIONIST

"How I Beat My Bloat"

When I accepted the position of nutrition director at *Prevention*, I moved to New York City from Tampa, Florida, but my husband, Jack, stayed behind for the first few months. Because Jack was still working in Florida part of every weekend, the only way we could see each other was if I flew back every Friday after work, returning Sunday night. I was a fairly frequent flyer before moving to New York, but nothing like this. For a few months, I spent at least six hours on a plane every weekend and believe me, my belly balked! I'd leave New York with a flat belly and go to bed Friday night looking three months pregnant. By the time my digestive system started to settle, I'd be at 30,000 feet again on Sunday night. Walking to work Monday morning, I'd feel self-conscious. After a few weeks of experimenting with the foods that ultimately became the Four-Day Anti-Bloat Jumpstart, I finally got a handle on my belly. I drank lots of water, traded my crisp, fresh apple for a few dried figs (less bulk), and swapped my peanuts for milder pumpkin or sunflower seeds. I also implemented a stress-reducing travel routine—relaxing music on my iPod, some deep breathing exercises, and a book I could get lost in—even when my flight was delayed three hours. It's amazing what a difference a few small changes can make!

—*Cynthia*

How Prone Is Your Belly to Bloat?

Discover how susceptible you are to belly bloat and water retention by taking this simple quiz. When you're finished, add up your score and compare to the ratings below:

QUESTION	A	B
Do you eat tend to eat too quickly? If yes, add 1 point for every speedy meal you eat per day (i.e., if you eat 4 times a day and they're all eaten at rapid speed, put a 4 in column A). If no, place a 1 in column B.		
Believe you are lactose intolerant? If yes, place a 1 in column A. If no, place a 1 in column B.		
Do you tend to talk a lot while you eat? If yes, place a 1 in column A. If no, place a 1 in column B.		
Do you add table salt to your food? If yes, add 1 point for every salt-sprinkled meal you eat per day (i.e., if you eat 4 times a day and you salt each meal, put a 4 in column A). If no, place a 1 in column B.		
Do you regularly binge on carbs? In other words, do you have episodes of eating more than you usually would of carb-rich foods at least once a week? If yes, add 1 point for every high-carb binge you can recall over the past week. If no, place a 1 in column B.		
Add 1 point to column A for each of the following foods you eat at least once a week: beans, lentils, nuts, cauliflower, broccoli, Brussels sprouts, cabbage, onions, peppers, raw citrus fruits. If you don't eat any of these foods at least once a week, add a 1 to column B.		
Do you chew gum, including sugarless? If yes, add 1 point for every piece of gum you chew per week (i.e., if you chew 1 piece a day, put a 7 in column A). If no, place a 1 in column B.		

QUESTION	A	B
Do you use sugar substitutes? If yes, add 1 point for every packet you use per day (i.e. if you use 2 in your morning coffee, place a 2 in column A). If no, place a 1 in column B.		
Do you eat sugar-free candies or sweets? If yes, add 1 point for every serving of sugar-free food you eat per week (i.e., if you suck on sugar-free candies in the afternoon at work M–F, place a 5 in column A). If no, place a 1 in column B.		
Do you suffer from sleep apnea? If yes, add 1 point. If no, place a 1 in column B.		
Do you eat fried foods? If yes, add 1 point for every serving of fried foods you eat per week (i.e., if you treat yourself to fries only once a week, place a 1 in column A). If no, place a 1 in column B.		
Do you drink carbonated beverages? If yes, add 1 point for every can or bottle you drink per week (i.e., if you drink 2 diet colas a day, place a 14 in column A). If no, place a 1 in column B.		
Do you drink coffee, tea, or acidic juice (orange or tomato) daily? If yes, add 1 point for every glass or mug you drink per week (i.e. if you drink 2 cups of coffee a day, place a 14 in column B). If no, place a 1 in column B.		
Would you rate your everyday stress level as high? If yes, place a 1 in column A, if no, place a 1 in column B.		
Add up your score in each column:	*TOTAL from column A:*	*TOTAL from column B:*

FINAL TOTAL (Subtract B score from A score): _____

If you scored:

A negative number: Congratulations! Your bloating risk is relatively low. You're already avoiding a lot of the foods and bad habits that contribute to excessive bloating and water retention. But that doesn't mean the Four-Day Anti-Bloat Jumpstart won't help you. You may not lose significant inches, but you will still *feel* lighter, healthier, and on a better path to long-term well-being.

0–5: Not so bad. You probably experience come-and-go bloat, what I like to call "bloat-flow"—one day you're swollen, a few days later, you've deflated again. The good news is that you can tame your tummy without making too many changes to your lifestyle. You should get some immediate gratification on the Four-Day Anti-Bloat Jumpstart.

5–10: You may experience a little withdrawal from your usual habits, but you'll be handsomely rewarded—you should experience a noticeable difference after just two days on the Jumpstart.

10+: Congratulations again! If you're confused, don't be. I say congratulations because you are perfectly suited to seeing fantastic results on the Four-Day Anti-Bloat Jumpstart, and therefore you're virtually primed for success on the Flat Belly Diet as a whole. That's because the Jumpstart itself is really a cleansing—of foods, drinks, and behaviors—that cause your body to unnecessarily hang onto fluid or produce excess gas and waste. It's not a detox, but it is a cleaner, simpler way to eat than you may be used to. And because of that, you're likely to see some major belly shrinkage.

A Thinner, Lighter You in Four Days!

For me, this is truly an exciting moment, to be able to reveal this fantastic, superfast, and superhealthy plan for you. You will not believe your eyes, as the inches evaporate and your clothing suddenly feels looser. No, it's not magic. It's basic science. The Four-Day Anti-Bloat Jumpstart literally abolishes the foods, beverages, and behaviors that cause your belly to pooch out. And—as a bonus—it provides guidelines for reducing the chances of ever feeling this way again.

As you experience this phase, remember that you're taking the first step of your journey toward a healthier lifestyle. It's not just a smaller dress size. Here's what you're really gaining, in a nutshell:

* An easy, safe, food-based solution for the body part you most want to change

* A more intense focus on your long-term health

* A reduced risk of heart disease, diabetes, and cancer

* A comprehensive understanding of what constitutes a healthy meal

* A more mindful approach to meals that virtually eliminates emotional eating

If you've tried other diets in the past, you're probably used to focusing first and foremost on the scale. This is one of the most important ways in which the Flat Belly Diet is different. In the last chapter, you learned how important your emotional state is to achieving success on any diet plan. Keeping your focus on you and your ultimate goal of lifelong good health and well-being will make these dietary changes practically effortless. Be mindful that, even as you add new foods and subtract less healthy ones as prescribed on the Flat Belly Diet, you're also taking critical steps toward better emotional health. Every time you eat a meal from this plan, you're making a commitment to yourself that transcends a weight-loss goal. You're giving yourself the tools to live longer and healthier and enjoy the life you imagine.

Remember: This Four-Day Anti-Bloat Jumpstart is designed to eliminate both bloating and water retention. Losing bloat is not the same as burning fat (we'll tackle *that* in the next chapter!), but it still creates a major change in your appearance and confidence level.

That's not to say you won't lose some serious pounds! And you'll start right now. If you follow the instructions provided for the next four days, we estimate that you can expect to lose as much as 7 pounds and up to 5¾ inches from your waist, hips, thighs, bust, and arms combined. *No sweat necessary.* That's right—no exercise is needed. I didn't make these numbers up. They are actual pounds lost, all calculated by an expert who weighed and measured our test panelists. Rest assured: This plan is proven and effective.

Four Days—What to Avoid

The Jumpstart is carefully designed to deflate your tummy and spur your body to release excess fluid. The following foods are off-limits for these four days only. You'll notice that most of them are considered "healthy," so they should still have a place in your shopping cart—just not during the first four days you're on the Flat Belly Diet.

Avoid:

The salt shaker, salt-based seasonings, and highly processed foods. Water is attracted to sodium, so when you take in higher than usual amounts of sodium, you'll temporarily retain more fluid—which contributes to a sluggish feeling, a puffy appearance, and extra water weight. Cutting back on sodium and boosting your water intake will help bring your body back into balance. It'll also help reduce your risks of hypertension and osteoporosis. If you find your food lacks flavor without a few shakes of salt, use the recommended salt-free seasonings.

Excess carbs. As a backup energy source, your muscles store a type of carbohydrate called glycogen. Every gram of glycogen is stored with about 3 grams of water. But unless you're running a marathon tomorrow, you don't need all this stockpiled fuel. Decrease your intake of high-carbohydrate foods such as pasta, bananas, bagels, and pretzels to temporarily train your body to access this stored fuel and burn it off. At the same time, you'll be draining off all that excess stored fluid.

Bulky raw foods. A half-cup serving of cooked carrots delivers the same nutrition as one cup raw, but it takes up less room in your GI tract. Eat only cooked vegetables, smaller portions of unsweetened dried fruit, and canned fruits in natural juice. This will allow you to meet your nutrient needs without expanding your GI tract with extra volume.

Gassy foods. Certain foods simply create more gas in your GI tract. They include legumes, cauliflower, broccoli, Brussels sprouts, cabbage, onions, peppers, and citrus fruits.

Chewing gum. You probably don't realize this, but when you chew gum, you swallow air. All that air gets trapped in your GI tract and causes pressure, bloating, and belly expansion.

Sugar alcohols. These sugar substitutes, which go by the names xylitol or maltitol, are often found in low-calorie or low-carb products like cookies, candy, and energy bars because they taste sweet. Like fiber, your GI tract can't absorb most of them. That's good for your calorie bottom line, but not so good for your belly. Sugar alcohols cause gas, abdominal distention, bloating, and diarrhea. Avoid them.

Fried foods. Fatty foods, especially the fried variety, are digested more slowly, causing you to feel heavy and bloated.

Spicy foods. Foods seasoned with black pepper, nutmeg, cloves, chili powder, hot sauces, onions, garlic, mustard, chili, barbecue sauce,

WHEN BLOATING GETS BAD

Bloating is a common condition, but in some cases, it can be a sign of a more serious health problem. It's time to see a doctor when:

- Your symptoms don't improve on the Four-Day Anti-Bloat Jumpstart.
- You're suffering from chronic constipation, diarrhea, nausea, or vomiting.
- You have persistent abdominal or rectal pain or heartburn.
- You've lost weight without trying.
- You have a fever you can't explain.
- There is blood in your urine.

horseradish, catsup, tomato sauce, or vinegar can all stimulate the release of stomach acid, which can cause irritation.

Carbonated drinks. Where do you think all those bubbles end up? In your belly!

Alcohol, coffee, tea, hot cocoa, and acidic fruit juices. Each of these high-acid beverages can irritate your GI tract, causing swelling.

Four Days—What to Do

Follow the Four-Day Meal Plan exactly. This includes four smaller meals, one of which is a refreshing smoothie. This reduces the amount of food in your digestive system at any one time, cuts back on the release of stomach acids, and gets your body used to a four-meal-a-day schedule (which you'll be following on the rest of the Flat Belly Diet).

Eat four meals a day. The Jumpstart includes fewer calories—about 1,200 daily—than you'll be eating on the rest of the Flat Belly Diet, which allows about 1,600 per day. Eating less for these four days reduces the amount of food in your GI tract at any one time, cuts back on the release of stomach acids, and gets your body used to a four-meal-a-day schedule.

You'll notice a few staples including sunflower seeds, flaxseed oil, string cheese, and carrots. There are three reasons you'll see these items appear repeatedly:

1) We tried to limit the amount of food you have to buy to get started—and ensure you'll eat it before it goes bad.

2) We wanted to deliver a lot of nutritional and bloat-free bang for the buck.

3) We chose foods that need no added salt or condiments to taste good, so you won't be tempted to reach for one of these potential bloat-promoters.

Drink one full recipe of Cynthia's signature Sassy Water each day. We call it Sassy because it's a heck of a lot perkier than plain old water, just like Cynthia herself! But the ingredients in here aren't just for flavor: The ginger also helps calm and soothe your GI tract. Even more important: The simple act of making this Sassy Water every day will serve as a reminder for these four days that life is a little bit different, that things are going to change. It will help you focus on the task ahead: Getting a flatter belly once and for all.

Sassy Water

```
 2 liters water (about 8½ cups)
 1 teaspoon freshly grated ginger
 1 medium cucumber, peeled and thinly sliced
 1 medium lemon, thinly sliced
12 small spearmint leaves
```

Combine all ingredients in a large pitcher and let flavors blend overnight. Drink the entire pitcher by the end of each day.

Take a quick 5-minute after-meal walk. Moving your body helps release air that has been trapped in your GI tract, relieving pressure and bloating. All it takes is a leisurely stroll around the block, inside your office building, or at the mall; a quick walk with your dog, a neighbor, or your family members after dinner—anything that just gets you moving for 5 minutes. You can walk for more than 5 if you like, but at least 5 minutes are needed to help get things moving inside your belly.

Eat slowly. When you eat fast, you take in large gulps of air, which get trapped in your digestive system and cause bloating (think of a balloon filled with extra mouthfuls of air). That may not have been behind your mother's admonishment, but nevertheless, taking your time will keep your belly flatter.

Work your mind. The first days of a diet are never easy, and these four days are no exception. I'm asking you to change how you eat, and to give up some of the foods you're used to eating (like salt, perhaps) or drinking (like coffee)—and perhaps imagine you can't live without. Of course it's going to be worth it in the end—it does work and you will see your belly shrink. But until you see that poof disappear, you'll need a mental tune-up. That's where my Mind Tricks come in.

Mind Tricks are a way of giving a meal importance, making it a special, you-focused moment. They'll help you stay mindful of what you're

>>> FAST FACT

One way to take up less space in your intestine is to be mindful of what you put into it. For example, 1 cup of grapes takes up four times as much space as eating ¼ cup of unsweetened raisins.

"My Personal Flat Belly Trick"

I am very prone to water retention. I'm drawn to salty foods more than sweet ones, and whenever I have an especially salty treat (movie popcorn, anyone?), I get "puffy" for at least a day after. So if I have an early-morning TV appearance, I'm extra careful about what I eat the night before—you can bet there's no soy sauce involved! Some of us are genetically more prone to this phenomenon than others—nothing you can do about that. Here are some things to keep in mind about water retention, whether it's a been a regular companion or occasional nuisance for you.

Remember, it's not fat! I once had a friend call me in a panic saying she'd gained 4 pounds in one day. I asked if she'd eaten all her usual meals plus an extra 14,000 calories—because that, my friends, is what you'd need to eat to gain 4 pounds of body fat in a day. She hadn't been bingeing, and I'm guessing you don't, either. So don't beat yourself up about that kind of weight gain. It's just water retention, and you'll lose it again.

Know your own body. Keeping a journal can help you track certain patterns. You might be more prone to water retention during a certain part of your menstrual cycle, and journaling will show you when and for how long you tend to hang onto that extra fluid.

Plan ahead. If you're going to be in your bathing suit or you just plain want to look your leanest, avoid salty foods for at least several days ahead of time. This is one kind of weight change you can control completely.

—Cynthia

eating and why. As you embark on the four days' worth of Mind Tricks—sixteen in all, one at every meal—you'll surely find some that are so appealing that you'll want to repeat them again and again. In fact, you should repeat your favorites until they become a ritual. I'm all for doing whatever it takes to make you feel special.

Your Four-Day Shopping List

Produce

2 pints grape tomatoes

1 pint (2 cups) fresh green beans (can also be frozen)

1 large red potato

10 oz bag baby carrots

Half pint (1 cup) crimini mushrooms

1 large yellow squash (can also be frozen)

4 medium cucumbers

4 medium lemons

Dairy

½ gallon skim milk

1 package light string cheese

Frozen Foods

10 oz bag frozen unsweetened blueberries

10 oz bag frozen unsweetened peaches

10 oz bag frozen unsweetened strawberries

Dry Goods

1 box unsweetened corn flakes

1 box Rice Krispies®

12 oz package instant Cream of Wheat®

1 box instant brown rice

24 oz jar unsweetened applesauce

8 oz can pineapple tidbits canned in pineapple juice

1 cup bulk (or 1 small package) roasted or raw unsalted sunflower seeds

8 oz bottle cold-pressed organic flaxseed oil

8 oz bottle olive oil

1 small package raisins

7 oz can Sunsweet® Ones Dried Plums

Spices

1–2 knuckles fresh grated ginger

2 bunches fresh spearmint leaves

Meat/Seafood

2 packages Applegate Farms® Antibiotic-free Honey Maple Turkey

¼ pound tilapia

⅓ pound boneless skinless chicken breast

¼ pound turkey breast cutlet

1 can chunk light tuna in water

Make It as You Like It

The Four-Day Jumpstart is built around mild-flavored foods that won't irritate your GI tract. But, if it's just too plain for your palate, you can add any of these approved salt-free seasonings:

* Original and Italian medley Mrs. Dash® salt-free seasoning blends

* Fresh or dried: basil, bay leaf, cinnamon, curry powder, dill, ginger, lemon or lime juice, marjoram, mint, oregano, paprika, pepper, rosemary, sage, tarragon, or thyme

* Aged balsamic vinegar (use in moderation: 1 Tbsp = 5 calories)

The Four-Day Anti-Bloat Menus

Breakfast Day 1

1 cup unsweetened cornflakes
1 cup skim milk*
½ cup unsweetened applesauce
½ cup roasted or raw unsalted sunflower seeds
Glass of Sassy Water

MIND TRICK: Say hello, sunshine! Enjoy breakfast near a sunny window. Morning sunlight has been shown to be a mood booster and will set your body's master clock for maximum all-day energy.

Lunch

4 oz Applegate Farms® Antibiotic-Free Honey Maple Turkey, rolled up
1 light string cheese
1 pint fresh grape tomatoes
Glass of Sassy Water

MIND TRICK: Put some color in your day. Before sitting down, arrange a few cut flowers in a vase and place it on the table. You're working hard on this diet. You deserve something special for your efforts.

Smoothie

Blueberry Smoothie: Place 1 cup skim milk and 1 cup frozen unsweetened blueberries in blender and blend for 1 minute. Transfer to glass, and stir in 1 Tbsp cold-pressed organic flaxseed oil.

MIND TRICK: Take a virtual, visual vacation. Put on some Hawaiian music while you're preparing your meal and transport yourself to a beach with lapping water and coconut palms. For a truly amazing experience, rub a little suntan oil on your hands and face and inhale deeply. Who cares if it's snowing outside? You're in Hawaii.

Dinner

1 cup fresh or frozen cooked green beans (steamed or microwaved)
4 oz grilled tilapia
½ cup roasted red potatoes drizzled with 1 tsp olive oil
Glass of Sassy Water

MIND TRICK: Resize your settings. Set your table with smaller plates and bowls. It'll make you feel like you have more food than you actually have.

*Use Lactaid® 100% Lactose-Free Fat Free Milk if you have even mild lactose intolerance.

Breakfast Day 2

1 cup Rice Krispies®
1 cup skim milk
¼ cup sunflower seeds
4 oz pineapple tidbits canned in juice
Glass of Sassy Water

MIND TRICK: Find a one-meal-only mantra. Pick a calming word or phrase, such as "I'm doing this diet for me." Repeat it after every bite.

Lunch

3 oz chunk light tuna in water
1 cup steamed or microwaved baby carrots
1 light string cheese
Glass of Sassy Water

MIND TRICK: Convert a friend. Invite a pal to have lunch with you today and explain your meal. Try to remember as many principles of the Jumpstart as possible. This will help you remember why you're doing this, even though it's such a departure from your normal routine.

Smoothie

Pineapple Smoothie: Place 1 cup skim milk, 4 oz canned pineapple tidbits in juice in blender, add a handful of ice, and whip for 1 minute. Transfer to glass, and stir in 1 Tbsp cold-pressed organic flaxseed oil.

MIND TRICK: Hang up some inspiration. Keep, say, your "skinny jeans" on a hanger in full view, so you pass them every day. They'll serve as a reminder of your ultimate weight loss goal. They *will* fit you again.

Dinner

1 cup fresh crimini mushrooms sautéed with 1 tsp olive oil
3 oz grilled chicken breast
½ cup steamed brown rice
Glass of Sassy Water

MIND TRICK: Sing while you prepare dinner. According to German researchers, you can enjoy up to a 240 percent immunity boost as well as an increase of anti-stress hormones simply by singing.

Breakfast

1 cup unsweetened cornflakes
1 cup skim milk
¼ cup sunflower seeds
2 Tbsp raisins
Glass of Sassy Water

MIND TRICK: Focus on your moment. This morning, eat your breakfast with no distraction—no radio, no morning show, no newspaper. Focus on the flavor of each bite.

Lunch

4 oz Applegate Farms® Antibiotic-free Honey Maple Turkey, rolled up
1 light string cheese
1 pint fresh grape tomatoes
Glass of Sassy Water

MIND TRICK: Bring in some bling. Serve your Sassy Water in the finest crystal glass you own. Make this your Flat Belly glass and use it at every meal.

Smoothie

Peach Smoothie: Place 1 cup skim milk and 1 cup frozen, unsweetened peaches in blender and blend for 1 minute. Transfer to glass, and stir in 2 tsp cold-pressed organic flaxseed oil.

MIND TRICK: Give thanks. Take a moment of gratitude for the food you are eating, the body you are nurturing, and the life you're enhancing. No need to get religious—it's perfectly okay to thank the peach farmer and your parents!

Dinner

1 cup fresh or frozen cooked green beans (steamed or microwaved)
3 oz grilled or baked turkey breast cutlet
½ cup roasted red potatoes drizzled with 1 tsp olive oil
Glass of Sassy Water

MIND TRICK: Think about yourself. Remember the list you compiled in Chapter 3, the one listing all the important people in your life? As you eat this meal, reflect on all you're doing to care for your body and your spirit.

Breakfast   Day 4

1 packet instant Cream of Wheat®
1 cup skim milk
¼ cup sunflower seeds
2 Sunsweet® Ones Dried Plums
Glass of Sassy Water

MIND TRICK: Laugh it up. A four-year-old laughs around 400 times a day. An adult, around 15. Today, even if you're alone when you sit down to your meal, laugh at your bowl of Cream of Wheat, howl at your glass of Sassy Water.

Lunch

4 oz Applegate Farms® Antibiotic-Free Honey Maple Turkey, rolled up
1 cup steamed or microwaved baby carrots
1 light string cheese
Glass of Sassy Water

MIND TRICK: Arrange your plate. Take a few minutes to prepare today's lunch with the flair of a gourmet chef. Wrap the turkey slices around the cheese and carrots, then slice on the bias and arrange. Garnish with a few sprigs of fresh herbs.

Smoothie

Strawberry Smoothie: Combine 1 cup skim milk and 1 cup frozen, unsweetened strawberries in blender. Blend, transfer to glass, and stir in 2 tsp cold-pressed organic flaxseed oil.

MIND TRICK: Before you sit down to eat, close your eyes and say something kind and reassuring about your body. Mention how much you love your arms or how people tell you you have great eyes or a fantastic smile.

Dinner

1 cup fresh or frozen yellow squash sautéed with 1 tsp olive oil
3 oz grilled chicken breast
½ cup steamed brown rice
Glass of Sassy Water

MIND TRICK: Serve today's dinner on your best china. Set a proper place setting with the good silver and the damask napkins.

Track Your Progress

Keeping a food journal is a research-proven way to help you commit to your new way of eating. Studies have continually shown that keeping a log of what you eat and how you feel while you're eating helps you stay on track with new lifestyle choices. In addition to being good for the soul, there is now increasing evidence to support the concept that journaling has a positive impact on physical well-being. University of Texas at Austin researcher James Pennebaker, PhD, has scientifically shown that regular journaling strengthens immune cells, called T-lymphocytes.[3] Other research indicates that journaling decreases the symptoms of asthma and rheumatoid arthritis. Pennebaker believes that writing about stressful events helps you come to terms with them, thus reducing the impact of these stressors on your *physical health*.

But in addition to all those things, keeping a journal is a simple way to feel as you're making significant progress. When I was training for my first (and only) marathon, I can honestly say that one of the biggest motivators in getting me into my running shoes and out the door every morning was my running log. All I wanted to do was fill that baby up, and I would get engrossed in watching the mileage accumulate week after week.

Similarly, your Flat Belly Diet Journal will inspire you to focus on and achieve your weight loss goals.

For the Four-Day Anti-Bloat Jumpstart, I'm going to give you a basic journal page that you can photocopy and carry with you. Later, when you complete the Jumpstart and begin the Flat Belly Diet, I'll ask you to spend a bit more time journaling about specific issues that you may have about food and your body confidence. For now, take these four days to get used to the format of the food journal—and start building the habit of sitting down and recording everything you've put into your mouth that day.

On the next page, you'll find a blank copy of the grid you'll be using for the next four days and instructions on using it. A few rules of the road:

1. Forget spelling and punctuation.

2. Write quickly to ward off your inner critic.

3. Speak from your heart.

The Jumpstart Journal

Day Number:				Date:

MEAL	HUNGER RATING AT MEAL START	MOOD	HUNGER RATING AT MEAL END	THOUGHTS/ OBSERVATIONS/ CHALLENGES
BREAKFAST				
LUNCH				
DINNER				

Instructions

Each day, you should:

* Fill in the DAY and DATE at the top of the grid.

* Enter a number under the HUNGER RATING AT MEAL START column. Documenting your hunger rating at the start of each meal lets you know which foods keep you satiated and which ones have you anticipating your next repast. Use the following scale:

    −5 = starving. You want to devour the first thing you see and have a hard time slowing down.

    −3 = overly hungry and irritable. You feel like you waited too long to eat.

    0 = mild to moderate hunger. You may have physical symptoms of hunger like a growling tummy and that "I need to eat soon" feeling, but you aren't starving or experiencing any unpleasant symptoms such as a headache, shaking, etc.

    3 = hunger but not craving-free. You're full, but you don't feel quite satisfied; your thoughts are still focused on food.

    5 = just right. Your hunger is gone and you feel satisfied. Your mind is off food, and you're ready to take on the next task. You feel energized.

    7 = a little too much. You think you overdid it. Your tummy feels stretched and uncomfortable. You feel kind of sluggish.

* Enter a description of your mood, being as descriptive as possible.

* Enter your THOUGHTS/OBSERVATIONS/CHALLENGES. For example, you feel energized, your clothes are getting looser, your skin is suddenly glowing. Or you could barely make it through for four hours. The idea is to give you a glimpse of how certain foods make you feel, and what food combinations seem to work best for you.

* Enter a number under the Hunger Rating at Meal End column, using the guide above.

Day Four and Beyond

As you reach the final day of your Anti-Bloat Jumpstart, I know what you're feeling. You're feeling lighter, stronger, more confident, and more self-centered (in a good way) than you've ever felt before. That's exactly where I want you to be, because that's exactly the right mind-set you need to be able to forge ahead and begin the next phase of the Flat Belly Diet: the 28-day program that will give you the tools to manage your health and maintain your desired goal weight for the rest of your life.

Questions Anyone?

Cynthia answers some of your most common and pressing queries

Q: *Is it important for me to measure my food?*
A: Yes. Measuring will help ensure that this carefully calculated plan gives you the results you're looking for. Without measuring, it's very easy to miscalculate and rack up hundreds of extra calories. I've certainly seen this in my practice as a registered dietitian. Always measure foods—especially those that pack a lot of calories in small amounts, including oil, nuts, seeds, peanut butter, avocado, pasta, rice, and oatmeal.

Measuring will also help you become more familiar with serving sizes. Studies show that most people underestimate serving sizes when eyeballing them—that can mean 20 to 40 percent more food (and calories). For cup and spoon measurements (½ cup, 1 Tbsp, etc.), be sure to level the top. Make sure you keep a good set of measuring cups and spoons on hand.

Q: *What does 3 ounces of meat look like?*
A: Three ounces of meat is about the thickness and width of a deck of cards. If you really want to be precise, you can use a food scale to weigh your meat (you can find these at most kitchen stores), or you can do a little label math. For example, a package of Applegate Farms® deli meat contains 7 ounces, so a 3-ounce serving is a little less than half the package.

Q: *You recommend I cook my carrots. How long do I microwave veggies? Do I need to add water?*

A: All microwaves vary, but most veggies take about 3 minutes per cup to "cook" in the microwave. You should not have to add water—just place your veggies in a microwave-safe dish, cover with waxed paper, and cook.

Q: *What is a calorie?*

A: A calorie is a unit of measurement of energy. Technically speaking, it's the energy needed to increase the temperature of 1 gram of water by 1°C. (Guess that's why dietitians take so much chemisty in college!) In everyday terms, it's energy that can have one of four origins, and one of three destinations. There are four sources of calories: carbohydrates, protein, fat, and alcohol. The first three types are essential to the body, but alcohol is not. When one of these types becomes available to the body, the cells will do one of three things with this energy. Basically, there is a priority system. Fuel is the #1 priority of every cell in the body. Just like cars need gasoline, cells need fuel to perform their jobs (breathing, circulation, movement, etc.). Carbohydrate calories are the cells' preferred source of energy. The next priority is repair, healing, and maintenance. Your body takes the energy from proteins and fats and uses them to patch up cells that are damaged or create new cells. Your muscles, bones, skin, and immune system rely on protein and fat energy for this work. And finally, if all the cells are properly fueled and repaired or replaced, your body takes the leftover or unneeded energy and stores it away in your fat cells. When your body is in "energy balance," it means the number of calories that showed up for work (the amount eaten) matched your needs perfectly. If you're in a positive energy balance, too many showed up and you end up storing some (i.e., weight gain); a negative energy balance means not enough calories are available. This can result in fatigue, feeling run down, and getting sick or injured. The Flat Belly Diet is designed to keep you in balance—it provides enough energy in the form of carbohydrates, proteins, and fats, but not too much.

The Flat Belly Diet Basics

CHAPTER 5

Wow.

Isn't it amazing how dramatically you can change the way you think and feel in just four short days? You've just completed a major milestone on the Flat Belly Diet—you've mastered the elusive art of eliminating water retention and bloat from your life forever. And, if you completed each Mind Trick, you've accumulated lots of little useful strategies you can employ anywhere, anytime, to boost your confidence and stay motivated. But now that you've seen how a flatter belly looks, and you've felt the renewed confidence that comes from experiencing such fast results, you're ready to move on to the next—and most important—piece of the Flat Belly Diet: You're ready to lose belly fat.

As I've said before, the Flat Belly Diet is different from any other diet

READ A FLAT BELLY
SUCCESS STORY

Donna Christiano
Age: 47
Pounds lost: 7 in 32 days
All-over inches lost: 6.5

"It's pretty amazing, when you think about it," exclaims Donna Christiano. "Seven pounds plus six and a half inches in a month—and never a day when I was hungry!" Donna calls the Flat Belly Diet the first weight-loss regimen she's followed that kept her satisfied 100 percent of the time. And she gives the MUFAs all the credit. "There's really something to them," she says. "I went away on vacation and stayed pretty true to the meal plan, but I couldn't always include a MUFA. And when I didn't, I found I was much hungrier than I thought I'd be."

But there's more, she adds. Since she started on this plan, she's become increasingly interested in doing what is good for her. In particular, she's much more conscious of eating healthy foods. She ate healthy food before, but supplemented it with a lot of junk. On one of her earlier diets, she explains, they gave you a certain number of points for what you ate and she'd "spend" 15 on junk and seven on what was good for her.

before

after

Not anymore. "I'm 47," she says, "I'm not getting any younger. This is the age when things start creeping up on you. So, for example, I used to love milk chocolate. Now, I've started eating only dark chocolate. I try to optimize what I'm eating, too.

Before, I put powdered creamer in my coffee, but now I realize that it's full of chemicals, so I've started using sweetened soymilk. I put cinnamon in coffee because it's another antioxidant. I add blueberries to my yogurt in an effort to get the biggest bang for the buck."

The best part, though, is that her belly is getting flatter. She relates a single anecdote that best illustrates her success: She attended an exercise class with her neighbor Roseanne, whom she describes as tiny, tiny, *and tiny*. "She has a tiny

NOW

waist, tiny hips. Just gorgeous. So we were in this class together, following along with the instructor, and I happened to glance in the mirror. I saw this woman with a really flat belly and I thought, oh, that's Roseanne behind me. Then I looked again. And I said to myself, 'Wait a minute! That person's wearing a red shirt. *I'm* wearing a red shirt. I think that's me!' And it *was*.

"This diet just works for me," she raves. "Everything about it. I'm a snacker, and I like to eat every four hours. That's part of the diet. I love peanut butter for breakfast, and I can have two tablespoons. Two tablespoons! It's practically *sliding* off the bread and I think, wow! This is so much food! And the Snack Pack? Come *on*! Chocolate chips with six ounces of light yogurt and a piece of fruit? Chocolate chips *on a diet*. Can you imagine?"

plan out there. Cut calories from anywhere in your diet and you will lose pounds. Add in cardiovascular exercise and strength training, and you will even lose body fat. But no other diet can target *belly fat specifically* the way this diet can. That's because the Flat Belly Diet contains a significant amount of MUFAs (aka monounsaturated fats). These unique fats—first brought to our attention by researchers studying the health benefits of the Mediterranean diet and lifestyle—are like little miracle workers in your belly. When you consume a reduced-calorie diet that's high in MUFAs, you will not only lose pounds. You will also lose visceral belly fat, the type of body fat that wraps around your internal organs, secretes inflammatory chemicals, and ups your risk of chronic disease. I know that you probably bought this book to lose your belly pooch so you can feel better about yourself and maybe even look better in your clothes. But succeeding on the Flat Belly Diet promises an even greater reward than that: a longer, healthier life.

Three Rules to Eat By

Over the next 28 days—and beyond—you are going to eat very well. How does Spicy Shrimp with Chili Bean Glaze sound? Chicago-Style Hot Dog, anyone? How about a Chocolate Chip Cherry Waffle? They're just a few of the anti-"diet" dishes you'll be eating. And it won't be a lot of work. We've developed two different ways to follow the Flat Belly Diet: The first, in Chapter 6, is perfect if you're too busy to even think about cooking dinner. It's also a great way to familiarize yourself with this new way of eating, because it lays everything out for you. You don't have to think about portion size at all because everything is pre-portioned. Chapter 7 is loaded with MUFA-packed recipes and meal additions that will allow you to follow the Flat Belly Diet when convenience foods may not be an

Did You Know ?

A 1-pound fat loss is something to celebrate—though not, of course, with a fattening treat! One pound of fat is the equivalent of 4 sticks of butter. Close your eyes and imagine 4 sticks of butter gone from your belly. This is what you can do for yourself!

option—family dinner night, for example, or when you're entertaining. Both plans adhere to three very important Flat Belly Diet rules that you must follow if you expect to reap the health and weight-loss rewards on this plan. They are:

* Rule #1: Eat a MUFA at every meal.

* Rule #2: Stick to 400 calories per meal.

* Rule #3: Never go more than four hours without eating.

If you remember nothing else from this book, remember those three rules. They're all you need to know to lose weight and keep it off. Before I explain each rule, though, I want to give you a little bit of history on how Cynthia created this plan. After all, she spent a decade studying nutrition science and public health. The Flat Belly Diet is an improvement on one of the healthiest diets in the world, the Mediterranean diet.

The Origins of the Flat Belly Diet

The Mediterranean diet has been the traditional way of eating in countries surrounding the Mediterranean Sea, including Greece, Israel, Spain, and Italy, for centuries. Please understand: The Mediterranean diet is not

(continued on page 94)

READ A FLAT BELLY
SUCCESS STORY

Kevin Martin
Age: 50
Pounds lost: 13.5
All-over inches lost: 11.25

"It's not like I didn't contribute to this belly," laments Kevin Martin. "I'm a supervisor. So I ride around all day in my truck. You know how that is. You spend your day eating lots and lots of stuff that's not good for you. I'd head out to work at 6 a.m., and I'd stop on the way and get my coffee and I might get two donuts to go with it. By nine, I'm getting a bacon, egg, and cheese sandwich. And a Snapple. That's breakfast. By twelve, I'm eating pizza or a big huge sandwich, and that holds me until two, when it's time for a couple of Funny Bones and a drink. At four, I get home and go straight for the cookies in the cabinet and then it's dinnertime." After dinner, it's poker on the computer. The next day? "Same thing all over again." After a long pause, he asks: Is it any wonder that spare tire around my waist was slowly inflating?

before   *after*

"I wanted to lose 12 to 15 pounds and get rid of the spare tire around my waist," says the 50-year-old, adding that he's never been on a diet before. Not successfully, anyway. He tried them several times with his wife but never stayed on one more than a couple of days.

This time, he says, was different. "I guess the timing was just right with this one. Summer was coming. And I wanted to be able to take off my shirt in public." He also knew he needed something to get him off the computer—playing online poker had become his nightly activity—and into the gym. "I belonged to a gym but never went.

I was paying all that money—for nothing. So because I was also on the (flat belly) exercise program, I started going to the gym again."

He started the diet and his summer vacation on the same day. He believes that made it easier for him since he was out of his truck, away from the places that he used to frequent, away from the Funny Bones and pizza parlors. "And the good thing was, we went away to an island, so the first thing I did in the morning was ride my bike the length of the island—which was almost 10 miles." That, he says, was something he never was able to do before.

Kevin admits that the first 4 days—the Anti-Bloat diet—were a challenge for him. Going cold turkey from coffee was hard enough, he recollects. But giving up all the

NOW

junk food? That was *really* hard for him. Still, he was committed. And he stuck to it. What kept him going was his athlete's sensibility. "I wanted to finish it. Get to day 32. I knew I would, too. I used to be a jock and I played all kinds of sports. When you're an athlete, you start something, you finish it."

After the first full week, he was amazed at how great he was beginning to feel. He is happy that he's doing something productive for himself *and* his body. Now when he gets home from work, instead of going for the cookies and the computer, he heads for the gym or takes a ride on his bike—or sometimes both. He has the energy now, he says.

And he's thrilled with his 13.5-pound weight loss. "I feel a lot better. I'm not tired ever. Or hungry. My main objective was to be able to take my shirt off in public and I'm there—now that I got rid of the fat. And with the gym, I'm working on tightening up my belly. Now that I've lost all this weight, I realize how terribly I had been treating my body. I won't be doing *that* again," he says. "Ever."

actually a single diet plan, per se, but rather *a smart and specific approach to eating* that has served these cultures well for thousands of years. A few foods figure prominently in the Mediterranean diet. They include:

* Olives and olive oil, almonds, and other nuts and seeds (all MUFAs)

* Locally grown, in-season fruits, vegetables, and legumes

* Whole grains

* Very limited portions of red meat

* Seafood several times a week

Hundreds of studies have linked this approach to a longer, more healthful life and a lower body weight. But the upside doesn't end there. Some of the latest scientific studies show that diets like the ones followed by Mediterranean peoples are also:

Better for Weight Loss

Researchers have learned that diets containing up to 40 percent fat are more effective at helping people lose weight and keep it off for life than low-fat diets containing less than 30 percent fat. The additional fat makes food taste better and boosts satisfaction—key factors whenever food's involved!

Better for Disease Prevention

Eating the way Mediterranean peoples do can help lower cholesterol levels, increase blood antioxidant levels, boost blood vessel flexibility, reduce risk of insulin resistance, metabolic syndrome, Alzheimer's disease, heart disease, and cancer.[1] Can't get much healthier than that!

How the Flat Belly Diet Is Different . . . and Better

The Flat Belly Diet is all this and more. What we've done here is taken the basic, scientifically proven principles of the Mediterranean diet and enhanced them by ensuring that you get a specific amount of a specific type of healthy fat—the MUFA—at every meal. We've also made it calorie-controlled, so weight loss is practically a no-brainer. And we've made it easier to incorporate the plan into your life, no matter how busy you are.

As I mentioned earlier, the Flat Belly Diet has just three rules to follow:

Rule #1: Eat a MUFA at Every Meal.

"A MUFA at every meal" has almost become a mantra for me. As you know, MUFA (MOO-fah) stands for monounsaturated fatty acid, a type of heart-healthy, disease-fighting, "good" fat found in foods like almonds, peanut butter, olive oil, avocados, even chocolate. MUFAs are an *un*saturated fat, and have the exact opposite effect of the unhealthy saturated and trans fats you've heard about in the news. Numerous

NOTES FROM OUR NUTRITIONIST

"Try My Favorite MUFA."

One of my favorite MUFAs is dry-roasted pumpkin seeds. I like to eat them one at a time. It's amazing how long it can take to eat two tablespoons when you eat them one after another vs. downing a handful at once. When I crack them between my teeth, I can sometimes feel the oil ooze out a little—that's because pumpkin seeds aren't as "meaty" as, say, almonds, so the oil is less dispersed throughout the seed.

—Cynthia

studies have shown that a diet rich in MUFAs is linked to a reduction in LDL cholesterol, the kind that clogs up arteries, and a boost in HDL, the kind that sweeps cholesterol out of the arteries and helps clear it from your body.

But there's more! MUFAs are delicious in and of themselves. Who doesn't love drizzling olive oil over a salad, or grabbing a handful of chocolate chips? You'll find the MUFA-rich foods on page 98 incorporated into the meal plans and Snack Packs. You can substitute one

How to Tell a Good Fat from a Bad One

Dietary fat is an important energy source. Used in the production of cell membranes and certain hormones, it's critical to the regulation of blood pressure, heart rate, blood vessel constriction, blood clotting, and the nervous system. Dietary fat aids the body in absorbing vitamins such as A, D, E, and K. But not all fats are created equal. Eating large amounts of the wrong kind of fat is very hazardous to your health. But telling good fats from bad fats isn't so easy, unless you know what to look for:

- **Monounsaturated fat** (MUFA) remains liquid at room temperature but may start to solidify in the refrigerator.

- **Polyunsaturated fat** remains in liquid form both at room temperature and in the refrigerator. Foods high in polyunsaturated fats include vegetable oils, such as safflower, corn, sunflower, soy, and cottonseed oils.

- **Omega-3 fatty acids** are a type of polyunsaturated fat found mostly in fat-rich seafoods such as salmon, mackerel, and herring. If you'd rather do your taxes than eat two fish meals a

MUFA for another as long as the calorie counts are equivalent. For example, you can exchange almond butter (202 calories) for macadamia nuts (203 calories).

The latest heart health guidelines from the National Institutes of Health advise that less than 7 percent of our total calories should come from saturated fat. Since the Flat Belly Diet is a 1,600-calorie plan, that equates to less than 12.5 grams of saturated fat a day. The following numbers will help you put that in perspective.

week, walnuts, flaxseeds, flaxseed oil, and, to a lesser degree, canola oil, also contain omega-3 fatty acids.

- **Saturated fats** become solid or semi-solid at room temperature. The marbling in red meat is one example, as is a stick of butter. Saturated fat is found mostly in animal foods, but three vegetable sources are also high in saturated fat: coconut oil, palm (or palm kernel) oil, and cocoa butter. Keep in mind that it's almost impossible to get your saturated fat intake down to zero. Even olive oil contains 2 grams of saturated fat per tablespoon.

- **Trans fats** raise LDL cholesterol and lower HDL cholesterol, increasing the risk of heart disease. They're quite possibly the most hated fats in all of fat-dom. Created when manufacturers hydrogenate liquid oils to increase their shelf life, they're found mostly in packaged products and nearly every food that contains shortening. Although nutrition facts labels must state trans fat content, the number is misleading, as manufacturers can legally claim 0 grams trans fats even if up to ½ gram per serving is present. Instead, look for the words "hydrogenated" or "partially hydrogenated" on ingredients lists to locate—and avoid—these deadly fats.

The grams of saturated fat in:

* ½ cup of premium chocolate chip ice cream = 12 (that means 48 per pint)

* 1 Tbsp of butter = 7 (that means 56 per stick)

* 1 cup (8 oz) of whole milk = 5 (that means 128 per gallon)

* 3 oz 85 percent lean ground beef = 5 (that means 25 per pound)

The main goal is not to eliminate saturated fat altogether, but rather to keep it in check and make most of your fat choices MUFAs.

PICK YOUR MUFA

FOOD	SERVING	CALORIES
SOYBEANS (EDAMAME), SHELLED AND BOILED	1 cup	298
SEMI-SWEET CHOCOLATE CHIPS	¼ cup	207
MACADAMIA NUTS	2 Tbsp	203
ALMOND BUTTER	2 Tbsp	202
PECANS	2 Tbsp	196
PINE NUTS	2 Tbsp	191
CASHEW BUTTER	2 Tbsp	188
NATURAL PEANUT BUTTER, CRUNCHY	2 Tbsp	188
NATURAL PEANUT BUTTER, SMOOTH	2 Tbsp	188
BRAZIL NUTS	2 Tbsp	186
SUNFLOWER SEED BUTTER	2 Tbsp	186
WALNUTS	2 Tbsp	185
HAZELNUTS	2 Tbsp	178
TAHINI (SESAME SEED PASTE)	2 Tbsp	178
PEANUTS	2 Tbsp	166
SUNFLOWER SEEDS	¼ cup	165
ALMONDS	2 Tbsp	164
CASHEWS	2 Tbsp	163

Rule #2: Stick to 400 Calories per Meal.

You've probably noticed from looking at the list of MUFAs that they're not exactly low-cal choices. They're all foods—nuts, oils, nut butters—that you're usually told to avoid when you're trying to lose weight. But because these MUFAs are so essential to losing belly fat, calorie control in what surrounds them takes on extra importance. All the meals in the Flat Belly Diet provide a MUFA *and* total about 400 calories. An added bonus of this controlled-calorie plan is that you can substitute one whole meal for another. You can eat breakfast for dinner

FOOD	SERVING	CALORIES
PISTACHIOS	2 Tbsp	161
PUMPKIN SEEDS	2 Tbsp	148
CANOLA OIL	1 Tbsp	124
SAFFLOWER OIL	1 Tbsp	120
SESAME OIL	1 Tbsp	120
SOYBEAN OIL	1 Tbsp	120
WALNUT OIL	1 Tbsp	120
FLAXSEED OIL	1 Tbsp	120
SUNFLOWER OIL	1 Tbsp	120
OLIVE OIL	1 Tbsp	119
PEANUT OIL	1 Tbsp	119
AVOCADO, CALIFORNIA (HAAS)	¼ cup	96
BLACK OLIVE TAPENADE	2 Tbsp	88
PESTO SAUCE	1 Tbsp	80
AVOCADO, FLORIDA	¼ cup	69
GREEN OLIVE TAPENADE	2 Tbsp	54
GREEN OLIVES	10 large	50
BLACK OLIVES	10 large	50

or lunch for breakfast. If you like, you can even eat four breakfast meals in one day. That's part of the ease of this plan. I don't expect that you'll love every single meal. But on the other hand, if you find a few you absolutely adore, it's perfectly okay to enjoy them to your heart's content.

Rule # 3: Never Go More than Four Hours without Eating.

I don't have to tell you that a diet won't work if it makes you feel hungry or tired. That's why on the Flat Belly Diet, you're *required* to eat every four hours. Waiting too long to eat can cause you to become so hungry (and irritable) that it's hard to even think clearly. That means you won't have the energy or patience to think through the healthiest meal choice, let alone prepare one. You'll probably want to tear into the first thing you see (bag of chips, handfuls of dry cereal straight from the box, cookies,

NOTES FROM OUR NUTRITIONIST

"Why Are Some MUFAs Liquid and Others Solid?"

People often ask me, "If MUFAs are liquid at room temperature, why are peanut butter, almond butter, and nuts solid?" The answer is because not all of what's in there is MUFA. The protein and fiber in nuts and nut butter make up a good percentage of their structure, and those are solid. If you look at the MUFA list, you'll notice that many of the foods are oils, which will indeed be liquid at room temperature, and the solid foods can be pressed to release their oils (think olive oil or almond oil).

—*Cynthia*

and so on) and you'll probably have a hard time slowing down while you eat and not reaching for seconds.

First up is breakfast—don't skip it. I know the temptation, but studies show that people who skip breakfast and eat fewer times during the day tend to be heavier than people who eat a healthy breakfast and eat three or four more times a day. This may be because people who skip meals tend to feel hungrier later in the day and then eat more than they normally would to compensate. It may also be that eating many small meals throughout the day helps people control their appetites.

Snacks are equally important, but when you eat them is entirely up to you. I like to have a snack in the evening while I'm reading manuscripts, but some of the editors I work with need a snack in the afternoon to keep them going until dinnertime. Your snacktime is entirely personal, and entirely essential. To help you include your snack every day, Cynthia has created a variety of Snack Packs that you can prepare ahead of time and take with you each morning. They're portable, and MUFA-loaded. Use the Snack Pack as a floating meal.

Snack Pack Options

There are 28 Snack Pack choices to choose from. You will see 10 sweet options, 10 savory options, 4 grab-and-go choices, and 4 smoothies. Choose any one you like. Just keep the following rules in mind:

1. You have *one* Snack Pack to "spend" per day.

2. Plan your Snack Pack in advance. I recommend carving out about ten minutes each night to think through your schedule for the following day. You should decide where in the day you'll "place" your Snack Pack based on what you have planned. You may need to pack it the night before and bring it with you so you'll have it ready when you need it.

3. You can eat the Snack Pack either between breakfast and lunch, between lunch and dinner, or between dinner and bedtime— whichever is best for your schedule. I just ask that you use it to ensure that you do not go more than four to five hours without eating. The goal is to use the Snack Pack to keep your energy and blood sugar steady, keep your metabolism revved up, and prevent your hunger from getting out of control (which often results in rebound overeating).

Sweet Snack Packs (10 combos):

Note: MUFA-rich items are in boldface.

1 packet plain instant hot oatmeal topped with 1 cup blueberries and 2 Tbsp **almonds**—324 calories

1 packet hot oatmeal topped with 1 cup raspberries and ¼ cup **chocolate chips**—367 calories

1 packet hot oatmeal topped with ½ cup (4 oz) canned pineapple and 2 Tbsp **macadamia nuts**—363 calories

2 Tbsp **peanut butter** swirled into 1 packet hot oatmeal and topped with 1 medium sliced apple—368 calories

1 medium apple cut into wedges with 2 Tbsp **peanut butter** as a dip, and 4 cups light microwaved popcorn—368 calories

½ cup (4 oz) canned pineapple mixed into ½ cup cottage cheese, sprinkled with 2 Tbsp **walnuts**—325 calories

1 cup sliced strawberries and ¼ cup **chocolate chips** mixed into ½ cup cottage cheese—347 calories

1 whole 100% whole wheat English muffin spread with 2 Tbsp **peanut butter,** topped with 1 medium sliced apple—388 calories

3 Ry Krisp® crackers spread with 2 Tbsp **almond butter,** topped or eaten with 1 medium sliced apple—387 calories

1 cup sliced strawberries and 2 Tbsp **peanuts** mixed into 6 oz (80-calorie) vanilla yogurt—366 calories

Savory Snack Packs (10 combos):

¼ cup hummus sprinkled with 2 Tbsp **pine nuts.** Eat as a dip with 1 cup red pepper slices– 331 calories

3 Ry Krisp® crackers spread with 2 Tbsp **black olive tapenade,** 1 cup grape tomatoes, and 4 oz rolled-up deli turkey slices—323 calories

½ cup canned, drained black beans, mashed, topped with ¼ cup **avocado,** chopped, and sprinkled with 1 chopped string cheese. Eat as a dip with 1 cup baby carrots—316 calories

½ cup canned, drained, mashed black beans, mixed with 1 cup halved grape tomatoes, topped with ¼ cup chopped **avocado** and sprinkled with 1 chopped string cheese and fresh cilantro (if you like). Eat as a spread with 3 Ry Krisp® crackers—401 calories

1 whole 100% whole wheat English muffin spread with 2 Tbsp **green olive tapenade,** topped with 4 oz deli turkey and 1 cup canned (water-packed) drained artichoke hearts—344 calories

1 toasted 100% whole wheat English muffin spread with ½ cup cottage cheese mixed with 1 cup halved grape tomatoes and sprinkled with 2 Tbsp **pine nuts**—421 calories

½ cup cottage cheese mixed with 1 cup chopped red pepper, 1 tsp salt-free Italian seasoning, and 10 sliced **large black olives.** Eat as a dip with 6 Ry Krisp® crackers—380 calories

4 oz deli turkey slices filled with ¼ cup hummus, sprinkled with 2 Tbsp **pine nuts,** and rolled up—391 calories

4 oz deli turkey slices filled with ¼ cup chopped **avocado,** 1 chopped string cheese, and 1 cup red pepper strips, and rolled up—316 calories

4 oz deli chicken slices filled with mixture of ½ cup cottage cheese and 1 Tbsp **pesto,** topped with 1 cup halved grape tomatoes and 1 cup canned (water-packed) drained artichoke hearts, and rolled up—360 calories

Grab & Go Snack Packs (4 combos):

1 string cheese, ½ cup (4 oz) pineapple fruit cup (in juice), 1 cup baby carrots, and 2 Tbsp **peanuts**—356 calories

1 string cheese, 4 cups popped light microwave popcorn, and 2 Tbsp **sunflower seeds**—345 calories

1 6 oz (80-calorie) yogurt, 1 medium apple, and 2 Tbsp **Brazil nuts**—346 calories

1 6 oz (80-calorie) yogurt, 1 medium orange, and 2 Tbsp **almonds**—314 calories

Smoothie Snack Packs (4 combos):

Put 1 cup skim or soy milk, 6 oz (80-calorie) vanilla yogurt, and 1 cup fresh blueberries plus a handful of ice OR 1 cup frozen blueberries in a blender. Blend for 1 minute, transfer to a glass, and stir in 1 Tbsp **flaxseed oil**—360 calories

Put ½ cup skim or soy milk, 6 oz (80-calorie) vanilla yogurt, ¼ cup **chocolate chips**, and 1 cup fresh raspberries plus a handful of ice OR 1 cup frozen raspberries in a blender. Blend for 1 minute, transfer to a glass, and eat with a spoon—387 calories

Put 1 cup skim or soy milk, one 6 oz (80-calorie) lemon yogurt, 1 medium orange peeled, cleaned, and sliced into sections, and a handful of ice in a blender. Blend for 1 minute, transfer to a glass, and stir in 1 Tbsp **flaxseed oil**—370 calories

Put ½ cup skim or soy milk, one 6 oz (80-calorie) vanilla yogurt, 1 tsp apple pie spice, 1 medium apple peeled and chopped, 2 Tbsp **cashew butter**, and a handful of ice in blender. Blend for 1 minute, transfer to a glass, and eat with a spoon—388 calories

 Log On for a Flatter Belly

At **www.flatbellydiet.com,** you can find everything you need to faithfully follow the entire Flat Belly Diet program for life. There, you can:

- Create your very own menu plans from hundreds of delicious MUFA-packed, calorie-controlled meals.
- Track your nutritional intake.
- Generate personal shopping lists.
- Read more about our success stories, whose profiles you see throughout this book, or nominate your own!
- Tap the experience, support, and motivation of hundreds of fellow Flat Belly dieters via message boards, blogs, and photo and video diaries.

www.flatbellydiet.com

CREATE YOUR OWN SNACK PACK

It's simple to create your own Snack Pack. Just remember to keep the total calorie count under 400. Include a selection from the MUFA list on page 98 with the following foods, recommended by Cynthia as super-healthy options, to round out the Packs. Share your favorite creations—and read others—at www.flatbellydiet.com.

GRAINS

Oatmeal—1 (1 oz) packet instant plain—100 calories

Popcorn—4 cups light microwave (a brand that provides 20–25 calories per cup popped, such as Wild Oats® organic plain popcorn, Smart Balance® Light, or Newman's Own® 94% fat free)—100 calories

Ry Krisp® crackers—3—75 calories

Thomas' 100% whole wheat English muffin—1 whole—120 calories

Frozen Lifestream Organic Flax Plus waffle—1—100 calories

Food For Life Ezekiel Sesame Sprouted Grain Bread—1 slice—80 calories

Food For Life Ezekiel Cinnamon Raisin Sprouted Grain Bread—1 slice—80 calories

Kashi 7 Whole Grain Puffs—1 cup—70 calories

Corn tortillas—2—90 calories

Dr. Praeger's frozen Homestyle Potato Pancakes—1—75 calories

Thomas' multigrain pita—½—70 calories

Uncle Ben's Ready Brown Rice—½ cup—110 calories

DAIRY

Cottage cheese, nonfat—½ cup—80 calories

Milk, skim or plain (unsweetened) soy—1 cup—80 calories

String cheese, light (1 oz)—80 calories

Yogurt, nonfat (6 oz)—80 calories

Feta cheese—1 oz—80 calories

Applegate Farms provolone cheese—1 slice—70 calories

Applegate Farms Monterey Jack with Jalapeño Peppers—1 slice—70 calories

Organic Valley Shredded Italian Four-Cheese Blend—¼ cup—90 calories

FRUITS

Apple, any variety, medium (size of a tennis ball)—80 calories

Berries (blueberries, raspberries, or strawberries)—1 cup—60 calories

Orange, medium—70 calories

Pineapple, canned in pineapple juice—4 oz or ½ cup—60 calories

Sliced banana—½ cup—70 calories

Pear—1 medium—100 calories

Red or green grapes—1 cup—60 calories

Kiwi—1 cup sliced—110 calories

Mango—1 cup sliced—110 calories

Papaya—1 cup cubed—55 calories

Peach—1 medium—50 calories

Plums—2 medium—60 calories

Watermelon—2 cups diced—90 calories

Mott's Natural Style Unsweetened Apple Sauce—1 cup—100 calories

Frozen Cascadian Farm Organic Pitted Dark Sweet Cherries—1 cup—100 calories

Unsweetened raisins—¼ cup—130 calories

VEGETABLES

Artichoke hearts, canned in water—1 cup—70 calories

Baby carrots—1 cup—50 calories

Grape tomatoes—1 cup—30 calories

Red (bell) pepper, sliced—1 cup—40 calories

Mann's Broccoli Coleslaw mix—12 ounce bag—50 calories

Organic mixed baby greens—2 cups—15 calories

Broccoli florets, raw—2 cups—40 calories

Cauliflower florets, raw—2 cups—50 calories

Radishes—1 cup sliced—20 calories

(continued)

CREATE YOUR OWN SNACK PACK (*cont.*)

Salsa—¼ cup—40 calories

Newman's Own Marinara Pasta Sauce—½ cup—60 calories

PROTEINS

Black beans, canned, drained—½ cup—90 calories

Hummus—¼ cup—100 calories

Deli chicken slices—4 oz—100 calories

Deli turkey slices—4 oz—100 calories

Applegate Farms uncured Black Forest ham—4 oz—100 calories

Gardenburger Black Bean Chipotle Veggie Burger—1—80 calories

Boca Original Vegan veggie burger—1—80 calories

Gardenburger Mama Mia veggie meatballs—6—110 calories

Chunk light tuna in water—3 oz—120 calories

Organic precooked chicken breast—3 oz—90 calories

Questions Anyone?

Cynthia answers some of your most common and pressing queries.

Q: *I like to eat! Does the Flat Belly Diet really let me eat as much as it appears to?*

A: Yes, it does. Remember, there are two stages to this plan. The 1,200-calorie Jumpstart only lasts four days. This initial stage is designed to help you lose your belly bloat and get your body and mind ready for the changes to come

The next 28 days provide four 400-calorie meals per day. In both stages, you're eating a breakfast, lunch, dinner, and a fourth meal called a Snack Pack. You can eat the Snack Pack between breakfast and lunch, between lunch and dinner, or between dinner and bedtime—whenever you need it most to keep hunger at bay. One caveat: It is essential is that you use your Snack Pack to ensure that you do not go more than four hours without eating. So, if, for example, you typically have breakfast at 8 a.m., lunch at noon, and dinner at 8 p.m., you need to eat the Snack Pack between lunch and dinner, as that is your longest stretch between meals. But, if you have breakfast as usual at 8 a.m. and lunch gets delayed until 3 p.m., better to have the Snack Pack around noon, and dinner at 7 or 8. Why? Because used this way, the Snack Pack will keep your energy and blood sugar steady, keep your metabolism revved up, and keep hunger at bay.

Q: *Why is the diet 1,600 calories per day?*

A: That's the number of daily calories it takes for a 40+ woman of average height, frame size, and activity level to get to and stay at her ideal body weight. So, 1,600 calories is not a starvation plan—it's enough to keep up your energy, support your immune system, and maintain your precious calorie-burning muscle. That means you won't feel run down, cranky, irritable, moody, or hungry. But you *also* won't be eating enough calories to hang on to your belly.

Q: *What do I do if I get hungry?*

A: I honestly don't think you will. Our test panel reported day after day that they never felt hungry. That's the magic of MUFAs and one of the benefits of the four-meal-a-day approach. But you might experience "false hunger"—when you think you're hungry, but the hunger is in your mind, not your body. This happens to many people when they change their eating patterns, especially if you're accustomed to overeating. Trust me, it doesn't last—false hunger fades as your body adjusts to your healthy new way of eating. True hunger is accompanied by physical symptoms—a growling tummy, for example. False hunger is more of an antsy, awkward feeling that originates above the neck. As part of the Flat Belly Diet, you will keep a food journal in which you'll rate your level of hunger and fullness before and after every meal. This, and filling in the column about your emotional state, will help you learn to differentiate between true and false hunger. If you feel that you are indeed experiencing physical hunger while following this plan, you can customize your plan by visiting flatbellydiet.com.

Q: *What about alcohol?*

A: Whether or not you drink on the Flat Belly Diet is up to you. As a health care professional, my goal has always been to help people make informed decisions that work best for their own lives. So here's the information I always share regarding alcohol: Current dietary guidelines recommend that if you don't drink, you should not start. In moderation, alcohol has been shown to lower the risk of heart disease, but it also carries risks. Just one drink a day is linked to an increased risk of breast cancer, and more-than-moderate drinking is tied to liver cirrhosis, high blood pressure, cancers of the upper gastrointestinal tract, stroke, injuries, and violence.

That said, most adults do consume alcohol, so if you do already drink, practice moderation, meaning one drink per day for women and up to two drinks per day for men. (One drink equals 12 ounces of regular beer, 5 ounces of wine, or 1.5 ounces (one shot) of 80-proof distilled spirits.) Each of these contains about 100 calories, so to stay on track with the Flat Belly Diet. You'll need to balance out those calories somehow. You can either burn 100 extra calories by exercising, or shave 25 calories from each of your four meals, or 50 from two. Taking 100 calories out of a single 400-calorie meal can leave you feeling too hungry, and since alcohol is an appetite stimulant, that could be a recipe for overeating.

Finally, of course, for health and safety, some people are advised not to consume alcoholic beverages at all, including pregnant and lactating women and individuals taking medications that can interact with alcohol.

The Four-Week Plan— Quick-and- Easy Meals

For just about everyone who's ever tried to lose weight, the word *diet* means long lists of forbidden foods, nonstop hunger, willpower struggles, and, eventually, a return to "normal" eating once you've met your goal— if you manage to struggle through and keep it. For Cynthia and me, *diet* has an altogether different meaning, one that's inspired by the National Institutes of Health, which simply defines diet as, "what a person eats and drinks; a type of eating plan." The Flat Belly Diet is a way of eating, one that allows you to get to, and then stay at, your ideal weight, while optimizing your health and energy and slashing your odds of getting nearly every chronic disease.

Our plan, as you know, has a specific goal: less belly fat. And less belly fat will, in turn, reduce your risk of disease. But even after we'd found the research supporting the notion that a particular food group—those beloved

MUFAs—could accomplish that, and even after Cynthia worked out the calorie counts and made sure that the nutrient requirements of the average woman could be met, we still had a bit of work to do. I knew that the Flat Belly Diet was going to have to compete with a whole shelf (or many shelves) full of popular plans, every one of them promising significant weight loss. I knew that to stand out on that shelf, it had to offer something—or many things—that other diets don't have.

Step one was asking *Prevention* readers what they loved and hated about traditional weight-loss diets. I quickly found that one woman's dietary nightmare is another's dream, which is probably why there's a diet book for every woman out there these days. Books exist for people with certain blood types, people who hate carbs, people with fat phobias, people who like, um, cabbage soup—whoever those unique and adventurous individuals might be. But I talked with Cynthia and learned a few universal truths about diets that work:

1. They offer sound advice and deliver on their promises. (Check. I would offer *Prevention* readers nothing less.)

2. They offer a plan that women can return to again and again, whenever their favorite jeans feel a little too snug. (Check. The Four-Day Anti-Bloat Jumpstart is an effective, safe solution you can turn to whenever you need an instant svelting.)

3. They are easy to live with. (Check . . . ?)

Ahhhh, that was the rub: How could we devise a plan that worked for everybody, all the time? I thought about this a long while and worried that it wasn't possible simply because there are as many definitions of "perfect" as there are readers of this book. Cynthia assured me, however, that it *was* possible! Her years of counseling dieters—and her rigorous planning for the Flat Belly Diet—are the backbone of this lifestyle. It was possible because the Flat Belly Diet offered:

* **Focus on health and energy.** Anyone can lose weight on a 1,200-calorie diet. But here's what you'll also lose: muscle, bone density, zest for living, sanity, and, if you follow a diet like that for too long, your sense of humor. (I've seen it happen!) Featuring healthy, wholesome foods and a 1,600-calorie-a-day guideline, the Flat Belly Diet is as healthy as they come.

* **Flavor.** It's food, after all! We consider no diet "complete" or "healthy" unless it's filled with delicious foods we love. This plan offers more taste than you can imagine.

* **Reality.** We wouldn't ask anyone to do something that we weren't willing—or able—to do ourselves.

* **Flexibility.** If you're pressed for time, you should be able to assemble meals quickly, with little or no cooking. But sometimes you might want to cook for your family or friends, and you should be able to do that without endangering your goal. Likewise, if you don't like a suggested meal, you should be able to swap it out for something you *do* want to eat. The Flat Belly Diet is about as flexible as it gets.

How It Works

Unlike most other diets, the Flat Belly Diet doesn't require you to follow a day-by-day, meal-by-meal menu. You will have a prescribed schedule of meals (four per day, including a snack), and a predetermined calorie count per meal and snack (roughly 400). Beyond that, we don't dictate

(continued on page 116)

READ A FLAT BELLY
SUCCESS STORY

"I'd had a bad couple of years and had put on extra weight
I just couldn't shake," says 52-year-old Patty Lloyd. "You really don't want to go down that road after 50, because it gets harder and harder to take it off. I knew something had to give."

Patty, who works in data processing and marketing, says the Flat Belly Diet couldn't have come at a more perfect time in her life. She was feeling out of control with her eating and spent all day sitting at a desk. "The only real exercise I got was cleaning the bathtub. The likelihood that a diet could help me turn this lethargy around and feel better in a short period of time was pretty slim. But I figured it was worth a try."

She loved the structure of the diet as well as the logic behind it because, as she explains, she does better when there is more to the guidelines than just food. Here she had to work out the timing of

before   *after*

four meals a day, follow a calorie count and, of course, learn a new concept she hadn't heard about before—eating a MUFA at every meal.

But the most surprising and welcome part of being on the Flat Belly Diet had to do with some pain she'd been experiencing. "I have bad arthritis in my knee," she explained, "and for some reason, after a week on the diet, my knee started feeling better." Wondering if there just might be a connection, she asked Cynthia, who explained that some of the MUFAs were anti-inflammatories and that might have had something to do with it. "Can you imagine eating food that can help with arthritis? I'll be happily *MUFAing* for the rest of my life!" Paty says.

Walking in general is much easier now. "My doctor told me that 1 pound of body weight is the equivalent of putting 10 pounds of pressure on your knee, so losing the weight combined with eating the anti-inflammatory MUFAs made great sense." She claims to *feel* younger, too. But what surprised her most was how *fast* it happened. She started feeling better almost immediately—even without losing a lot of weight.

NOW

"Sometimes dieting is discouraging because if you need to lose 20 pounds, it takes you a long time to start seeing results. I didn't lose all that quickly, but I felt markedly better. Which is a lot more important than any number on a scale."

Patty claims her favorite part of the food plan is eating peanut butter without guilt. Every morning she slathers 2 tablespoons of peanut butter onto a toasted English muffin and can't believe she's doing it. "Two tablespoons! Plus fruit. It's awesome," she exclaims. "On most diets, the breakfast is so skimpy. You look longingly at someone else's bagel and you think, *Oh, God. Someday I'm going to let myself go and have one of those.* But on this diet, it's not like that. The food doesn't make you feel like you're being punished. It tastes so good, and there's so much of it, you feel like you're eating just like everyone else." Even drinking the Sassy Water feels healthy, she comments. "To know you're doing something so good for yourself, *plus* you're not depriving yourself in any way—now really, what more can you ask from a diet?"

what to eat when. Instead, we offer suggestions—lots of them. In addition, *all of the meals are interchangeable*, so you can mix-and-match all you want. Our test panelists happily reported that this freedom of choice made it a breeze for them to follow the plan faithfully—even beyond the four-week test period.

You will eat four 400-calorie meals each day: three meals plus one Snack Pack (see Chapter 5 for suggested Snack Packs). Meals are categorized here as breakfast, lunch, and dinner, but because every single one follows the Flat Belly "400 calories with a MUFA" rule, you can shuffle them however you like. If you want pineapple-ham pizza for breakfast and apple-cinnamon waffles for dinner, go for it! There are 28 meals to choose from in each category, so, if you like, you can go for maximum variety and have something different for every meal, every day, for four weeks. On the other hand, if you find one breakfast you love and want to make it part of you morning routine every day, that's fine, too. (Join

FLAT BELLY DIET FUNDAMENTALS

- Pick any three Quick-and-Easy meals and one Snack Pack (from the list in Chapter 5) per day. Remember, it's okay to select a lunch meal for dinner, choose a dinner for breakfast, or eat the same one meal you love every day for lunch—the choice is yours.
- If you love to cook, or when you have time to cook, choose one serving of any recipe from Chapter 7 in place of any Quick-and-Easy meal.
- If you're on the run, choose one of the packaged options from the list of Flat Belly Ready-Made Meals at the end of this chapter.

the creature-of-habit club. I've eaten the same breakfast every day for three years!) For leisurely days when you have more time on your hands and feel like cooking, turn to Chapter 7, where you'll find more than 80 fabulous Flat Belly Diet recipes.

Wondering what you'll do when you don't even have time to slap together a sandwich? Have no fear: At the end of this chapter is a list of 59 Ready-Made Meals, including meal replacement bars, healthy frozen dinners, and even in-a-pinch fast-food options you can pair with a MUFA.

>>> FAST FACT

Being overweight or obese can cause cancer, shows a new study by researchers at the University of Oxford. Scientists studied more than 1 million British women, looking at the relationship between BMI and cancer. Obese and overweight women were twice as prone to developing endometrial cancer and cancer of the esophagus than women of normal weight. They also had a 53% greater risk of developing kidney cancer and a 24% greater risk of developing pancreatic cancer.[1]

Breakfast

Here are 28 tasty and, more importantly, filling ways to start your day. Among our testers—and their families!—the Cherry-Chocolate Waffle on page 120 was a huge hit. Whether sweet or savory is your breakfast of choice, you'll find plenty of great options here. MUFAs are in boldface.

Apple-Almond Oatmeal: ½ cup dry Quaker® Old Fashioned Quick 1-Minute Oats (150) (cooked with water to consistency of your choice), mixed with 1 medium apple, sliced (80), and sprinkled with apple pie spice and 2 Tbsp **almonds** (164)

Total Calories = 394

Apple-Cinnamon Waffle: 1 LifeStream® Organic FlaxPlus® frozen waffle, toasted (100), topped with 1 cup Mott's® Natural Style Unsweetened Apple Sauce (100), and sprinkled with cinnamon, nutmeg, and 2 Tbsp **walnuts** (185)

Total Calories = 385

Avocado-Tomato Herbed Breakfast Tacos: 4 6-inch corn tortillas, warmed (180); spread with 2 Laughing Cow® Light Garlic & Herb Wedges (70) and filled evenly with ½ cup Organic Valley® 100% Egg Whites scrambled with cooking spray (50) and 4 fresh basil leaves (0); sprinkle with 1 fresh sliced plum tomato (12) and ¼ cup **sliced avocado** (96)

Total Calories = 408

Banana-Pecan Oatmeal: ½ cup dry Quaker® Old Fashioned Quick 1-Minute Oats (cooked with water to consistency of your choice) (150), mixed with ½ cup sliced banana (70), and sprinkled with cinnamon, nutmeg, and 2 Tbsp **pecans** (196)

Total Calories = 416

Banana Split Oatmeal: Cook ½ cup dry Quaker® Old Fashioned Quick 1-Minute Oats (cooked with water to consistency of your choice) (150), mixed

with ¼ cup microwaved frozen strawberries (20) and topped with ¼ cup sliced banana (35), 1 Tbsp semi-sweet chocolate chips (50), and 2 Tbsp **peanuts** (166)

Total Calories = 421

Banana Waffle: 1 LifeStream® Organic FlaxPlus® frozen waffle, toasted (100), topped with ½ cup sliced banana (70) and sprinkled with cinnamon and nutmeg and 2 Tbsp **pecans** (196)

Total Calories = 366

Blueberry Nut Oatmeal: ½ cup dry Quaker® Old Fashioned Quick 1-Minute Oats (cooked with water to consistency of your choice) (150), mixed with 1 cup Cascadian Farm® organic frozen blueberries, warmed in microwave for 1 minute (70), and 2 Tbsp **cashews** (163)

Total Calories = 383

NOTES FROM OUR NUTRITIONIST

"Why So Many Calorie Counts?"

The numbers in the parentheses correspond to the calorie content of each ingredient. I provide them for a few reasons: First, to help you become familiar with the calorie levels of various ingredients—you may be surprised to find out just how many or few calories there are in certain foods. The second reason is to help you customize the plan. If you dislike a certain ingredient, don't have the same brand on hand, want to use up something you already have, or just want to experiment with a different way of preparing a meal, you can. Just be sure the food you added provides about the same number of calories as the one you took away. Use the Nutrition Facts label information to check the calorie content of packaged foods and for fresh foods, you can check the USDA database at www.nal.usda.gov/fnic/foodcomp/search/ or www.flatbellydiet.com.

—Cynthia

Breakfast BLT: 1 Thomas'® 100% Whole Wheat English Muffin (120) spread with 2 Tbsp **black olive tapenade** (88), and topped with ½ fresh plum tomato, sliced (6), 3 large Romaine lettuce leaves (3), 2 slices Applegate Farms® cooked organic turkey bacon (60), and 1 slice Applegate Farms® Organic Muenster Käse Cheese (85)

Total Calories = 362

Breakfast Tacos: 4 6-inch corn tortillas, warmed (180), filled evenly with 4 scrambled egg whites (½ cup Organic Valley® 100% Egg Whites makes about 1 cup scrambled eggs) (50), ½ cup fresh baby spinach leaves (3), ¼ cup salsa (40), and ¼ cup **sliced avocado** (96)

Total Calories = 369

Cashew Crunch: 1 slice Food For Life® Ezekiel 4:9® Sesame Sprouted Bread, toasted (80), spread with 2 Tbsp **cashew butter** (188), and sprinkled with ¼ cup raisins (130)

Total Calories = 398

Cherry-Chocolate Waffle: 1 LifeStream® Organic FlaxPlus® frozen waffle (100) topped with 1 cup frozen Cascadian Farm® Organic Pitted Dark Sweet Cherries, thawed (90), sprinkled with nutmeg and ¼ cup **semi-sweet chocolate chips** (207)

Total Calories = 397

Cinnamon Raisin Toast: 1 slice Food For Life® Ezekiel 4:9® Cinnamon Raisin Sprouted Bread, toasted (80), spread with ¼ cup nonfat ricotta cheese (50) topped with 2 Tbsp **walnuts** (185); and 1 medium apple (80)

Total Calories = 395

Dijon Egg Sandwich: ½ cup Organic Valley® 100% Egg Whites (50) scrambled in cooking oil spray with ¼ cup sliced red onion (23), dressed with 1 Tbsp Annie's Naturals® Organic Dijon Mustard (0), 1 slice Applegate Farms® Organic Muenster Käse Cheese (85), half a fresh plum tomato, sliced (6), ¼ cup

fresh baby spinach leaves (1), and ¼ cup **sliced avocado** (96), layered on
1 Thomas'® 100% Whole Wheat English Muffin (120)

Total Calories = 381

Farmer's Breakfast: 2 Dr. Praeger's® frozen Homestyle Potato Pancakes
(150) browned in pan with 1 Tbsp **safflower oil** (120); 2 slices cooked Applegate
Farms® organic turkey bacon (60), and 1 cup skim milk (80)

Total Calories = 410

Fruit & Nut Cereal: 1 cup Kashi® 7 Whole Grain Puffs (70) with 1 cup
skim milk (80), 2 Tbsp **almonds** (164), and 6 dried apricots (74)

Total Calories = 388

Mediterranean BLT: 1 Thomas'® 100% Whole Wheat English Muffin
(120), spread on one half with 2 Tbsp **black olive tapenade** (88) and the other
with one Laughing Cow® Mini Babybel® cheese (70); add ¼ cup sliced cucumber
(5), 3 sundried tomatoes jarred in olive oil (30), 3 large Romaine leaves (3), and
2 slices cooked Applegate Farms® organic turkey bacon (60)

Total Calories = 376

Muesli & Yogurt: 1 cup Kashi® 7 Whole Grain Puffs (70) mixed with 1 6 oz
Stonyfield Farm® Fat Free French Vanilla Yogurt (130), and 2 Tbsp **almonds**
(164); and 1 cup seedless red grapes (40)

Total Calories = 404

PB & B: 1 Thomas'® 100% Whole Wheat English Muffin toasted (120), spread
with 2 Tbsp **peanut butter** (188) and topped with ½ cup sliced banana (70)

Total Calories = 378

Peachy Pecan Oatmeal: ½ cup dry Quaker® Old Fashioned Quick 1-
Minute Oats (cooked with water to consistency of your choice in microwave for 1
minute) (150), mixed with 1 cup Cascadian Farm® Organic Sliced Peaches, thawed
(60), sprinkled with nutmeg and 2 Tbsp **pecans** (196)

Total Calories = 406

Peanut Butter Banana Toast: 1 slice Food For Life® Ezekiel 4:9®

Sesame Sprouted Bread, toasted (80), spread with 2 Tbsp **natural creamy peanut butter** (200), topped with ½ cup sliced banana (70); and 1 cup skim milk (80)

Total Calories = 430

Peanut Butter Toast & Yogurt: 1 slice Food For Life® Ezekiel 4:9®

Sprouted Sesame Bread, toasted (80), spread with 2 Tbsp **natural creamy peanut butter** (200) and 1 Stonyfield Farm® Organic Lowfat Maple Vanilla Yogurt (130)

Total Calories = 410

Pecan Raisin Cereal: 1 cup Kashi® 7 Whole Grain Puffs (70) with 1 cup skim

milk (80), sprinkled with 2 Tbsp **pecans** (196) and 2 Tbsp raisins (65)

Total Calories = 411

Potato Pancakes I: 2 Dr. Praeger's® frozen Homestyle Potato Pancakes

(150) browned in pan with 1 Tbsp **safflower oil** (120), ½ cup liquid Organic Valley® 100% Egg Whites (50) scrambled with ¼ cup sliced red onion (23) and half a fresh plum tomato, chopped (6); and ½ cup 100% orange juice (55)

Total Calories = 404

Potato Pancakes II: 2 Dr. Praeger's® frozen Homestyle Potato Pancakes

(150) browned in pan with 1 Tbsp **safflower oil** (120), ½ cup liquid Organic Valley® 100% Egg Whites (50) scrambled with ¼ cup fresh chopped red bell peppers (10) and 2 Tbsp chopped scallions (4), and ½ cup 100% orange juice (55)

Total Calories = 389

Raisin Almond Toast: 1 slice Food For Life® Ezekiel 4:9® Cinnamon

Raisin Sprouted Bread, toasted (80), spread with 2 Tbsp **almond butter** (202); and 1 cup skim milk (80) and ½ cup 100% orange juice (55)

Total Calories = 417

Toasted Egg-and-Cheese Sandwich: 2 slices Fit for Life®

Ezekiel 4:9® Sesame Sprouted Bread, toasted (160), spread with 1 Laughing Cow® Light Garlic & Herb Wedge (35), filled with omelet-style egg (½ cup

Organic Valley® 100% Egg Whites) (50) cooked in pan with cooking spray with ¼ cup sliced red onion (23) dressed with half of a fresh sliced plum tomato (6), 3 large Romaine lettuce leaves (3), and ¼ cup **sliced avocado** (96)

Total Calories = 373

Tropical Waffle: 1 LifeStream® Organic FlaxPlus® frozen waffle, toasted (100), topped with ½ cup drained pineapple tidbits packed in juice (60), and sprinkled with cinnamon, nutmeg, and 2 Tbsp **macadamia nuts** (203)

Total Calories = 363

Vanilla Macadamia Parfait: 1 cup Kashi® 7 Whole Grain Puffs (70) mixed with 1 container Stonyfield Farm® Fat Free French Vanilla Yogurt (140) and 2 Tbsp **macadamia nuts** (161)

Total Calories = 371

NOTES FROM OUR NUTRITIONIST

"Don't Even Think about Skipping Breakfast!"

When I was a dietitian in private practice, at least once a week someone would tell me that they "do better" when they skip breakfast. Unfortunately, this isn't true for anybody, and research proves it. In fact, a whopping 78 percent of successful dieters registered with the National Weight Control registry, a database of individuals who've lost 30 pounds or more and have kept it off for at least a year, eat breakfast. What about the theory that skipping this meal is a natural way to eliminate calories? Studies show that breakfast skippers make up for those calories by unknowingly eating more later in the day. Some of my clients swore that eating breakfast made them hungrier. Well, in fact, eating breakfast does stimulate your appetite because it kicks your metabolism into high gear. A faster metabolism means a flatter belly and more calories burned all day long, so you're better off with breakfast.

—Cynthia

Lunch

You're sure to find a delicious Flat Belly Diet spin on your favorite brown-bag standby here. I know I did: the Dijon Turkey Wrap on the next page. MUFAs are in boldface.

Boca Tacos: 4 6-inch corn tortillas, warmed (180), filled evenly with a ½ cup Boca Ground Burger Crumbles, microwaved (60), topped with ½ cup fresh baby spinach leaves (3), ¼ cup salsa (40) and ¼ cup **sliced avocado** (96)

Total Calories = 379

California Burger: 1 Boca® Original Vegan Veggie Burger (80) on 1 Food For Life® Ezekiel 4:9® Sprouted Burger Bun (150) dressed with 1 Tbsp Annie's Naturals® Organic Dijon Mustard (0), 3 large Romaine lettuce leaves (3), ½ cup Roland® Roasted Red Peppers (jarred in water) (30), and ¼ cup **sliced avocado** (96)

Total Calories = 359

Chicken Lettuce Wraps I: 3 oz organic grilled chicken breast (90), glazed with 1 Tbsp China Blue® Scallion Ginger Glaze (40), wrapped in 4 large Romaine lettuce leaves (4). Side of ½ cup fresh snow peas (20) with 2 Tbsp hummus (50) sprinkled with 2 Tbsp **pine nuts** (191), for dipping

Total Calories = 395

Chicken Lettuce Wraps II: 3 oz organic grilled chicken breast (90), chilled, brushed with 1 Tbsp China Blue® Scallion Ginger Glaze (40) wrapped in 4 large Romaine lettuce leaves (4); serve with ½ cup fresh snow peas (20) and 2 Tbsp hummus (50) sprinkled with 2 Tbsp **pine nuts** (191), for dipping

Total Calories = 395

Cheesy Spinach Ziti: ¼ cup cooked whole wheat penne (105), tossed with 1 Tbsp **extra virgin olive oil** (119), ¼ cup nonfat ricotta cheese (50), 2 Tbsp Organic Valley® Shredded Italian Four-Cheese Blend (45), ½ cup fresh baby spinach leaves (3), 2 Tbsp sliced onions (6), and ½ cup Newman's Own® Marinara Pasta Sauce (60)

Total Calories = 388

Chilled Chicken Pasta: ¼ cup cooked and chilled whole wheat penne (105) tossed with 1 Tbsp **pesto sauce** (80), 3 oz organic pre-cooked chicken breast, diced (90), 1 cup grape tomatoes, halved (30), ¾ cup shredded carrots (38), and 2 Tbsp Organic Valley® Shredded Italian Four-Cheese Blend (45)

Total Calories = 388

Chilled Spicy Italian Sausage Pasta: 1 Applegate Farms® Organic Sweet Italian sausage, cooked and chopped (150), tossed with ¼ cup cooked whole wheat penne, chilled (105), 1 cup grape tomatoes, halved (30), ¾ cup shredded carrots (38), and ¼ cup chopped celery (5) with 1 Tbsp **pesto sauce** (80)

Total Calories = 408

Crunchy Tuna Melt: 1 slice Food For Life® Ezekiel 4:9® Sesame Sprouted Bread (80) topped with 2 oz chunk light water-packed tuna (80), 2 Tbsp **sunflower seeds** (165), and 1 slice Applegate Farms provolone cheese (70), and placed under broiler or in toaster oven to melt

Total Calories = 395

Dijon Turkey Wrap: 1 Thomas'® Whole Wheat Sahara wrap (170) spread with 1 Tbsp Annie's Naturals® Organic Dijon Mustard (0), sprinkled with 2 Tbsp **pumpkin seeds** (148) and filled with 2 oz Applegate Farms® Antibiotic-free Honey Maple Turkey (50), ¼ cup sliced red onion (23), half of a fresh plum tomato, sliced (6), and 3 large Romaine lettuce leaves (3)

Total Calories = 400

Dipping Trio: ⅔ cup frozen Cascadian Farm® Organic Edamame, thawed (120), dressed in 1 Tbsp Annie's Naturals® Goddess Dressing (45); 2 Ryvita® Dark Rye Crispbread crackers (70); ½ cup organic baby carrots (25) with 2 Tbsp **tahini sauce** (178) for dipping

Total Calories = 438

Exotic Turkey Roll-Ups: 3 oz Applegate Farms® Antibiotic-free Smoked Turkey slices (75) wrapped around 1 oz (2 Tbsp) of Sabra™ Babaganoush

(80), ½ cup sliced Roland® Roasted Red Peppers (jarred in water) (30), and 2 Tbsp **pine nuts** (191)

Total Calories = 376

Ham & Bleu Cheese Salad: 2 cups organic mixed baby greens (15)

tossed with 2 Tbsp Annie's Naturals® Goddess Dressing (90), topped with half of a fresh plum tomato, sliced (6), 3 oz Applegate Farms® uncured Black Forest ham, chopped (75), 2 Tbsp crumbled gorgonzola (50), and 2 Tbsp **pumpkin seeds** (148)

Total Calories = 384

Italian Sausage Wraps: Sauté in 1 Tbsp **canola oil** (124): 1 Applegate

Farms® Organic Sweet Italian sausage, chopped (150), ½ cup fresh chopped bell pepper (20), and ½ cup sliced red onion (46); distribute evenly onto 4 large Romaine leaves (4), sprinkle with 2 Tbsp crumbled gorgonzola (50), and roll up

Total Calories = 394

Meatball Melt: 1 Thomas'® Multigrain Pita (140) filled with 3

Gardenburger® Mama Mia Veggie Meatballs (55) and 2 Tbsp Organic Valley® Shredded Italian Four-Cheese Blend (45). Drizzle with 1 Tbsp **extra virgin olive oil** (119). Place under broiler or in toaster oven to toast pita and melt cheese. Serve with ½ cup Newman's Own® Marinara Pasta Sauce (60) for dipping

Total Calories = 419

Mediterranean Wrap: 1 Thomas'® Whole Wheat Sahara wrap (170)

spread with 2 Tbsp **black olive tapenade** (88), filled with 2 oz turkey pastrami (60) ¼ cup sliced red onion (23), half of a fresh plum tomato, sliced (6), and 3 large Romaine lettuce leaves (3); 1½ cups red grapes (60)

Total Calories = 410

Muffuletta Wrap: 1 Thomas'® Whole Wheat Sahara wrap (170) spread

with 2 Tbsp **black olive tapenade** (88), and filled with 2 oz Applegate Farms® Antibiotic-free Honey Maple Turkey (50), 1 slice Applegate Farms® provolone cheese (70), ¼ cup sliced red onion (23), ¼ cup chopped celery (5), and 3 large Romaine lettuce leaves (3)

Total Calories = 409

Niçoise Salad: Toss 2 cups organic mixed baby greens (15) with 2 Tbsp Annie's Naturals® Organic Dijon Mustard to coat (0). Top with 1 cup skin-on red potatoes, cubed, boiled, and chilled (100), 10 sliced **large black olives** (50), ½ cup chopped green beans (15), ¼ cup chopped celery (5), ½ cup grape tomatoes, halved (15) and 4 oz chunk light water-packed tuna (160)

Total Calories = 360

Pesto Ham & Cheese Sandwich: 1 Thomas'® 100% Whole Wheat English Muffin (120) spread with 1 Tbsp **pesto sauce** (80), filled with 4 oz Applegate Farms uncured Black Forest ham (100), half of a fresh plum tomato, sliced (6), 3 large Romaine leaves (3), and 1 slice Applegate Farms provolone cheese (70); 1 cup grape tomatoes (30)

Total Calories = 409

Picnic Lunch: 4 Ryvita® Dark Rye Crispbread crackers (140) spread with 2 Tbsp Annie's Naturals® Organic Dijon Mustard (0), with 13 slices of Lightlife® Smart Deli Pepperoni (70), 10 **large green olives** (50), and ½ cup organic baby carrots (25) with ¼ cup hummus (100) for dipping

Total Calories = 385

Shrimp Lettuce Wraps: 4 large Romaine lettuce leaves (4) filled evenly with 3 oz medium shrimp (90), glazed with 1 Tbsp China Blue® Scallion Ginger Glaze (40), broiled, chilled, and tossed with ¼ cup chopped celery (5), 2 Tbsp minced red onion (12), ¼ cup fresh chopped red bell peppers (10), and 2 Tbsp **cashews** (163)

Total Calories = 324

Southwest Pita Melt: 1 Thomas'® Multigrain Pita (140) filled with 1 slice Applegate Farms® Monterey Jack with Jalapeño Peppers (70) and 1 Gardenburger® Black Bean Chipotle Veggie Burger (80), defrosted in the microwave. Place in toaster oven to brown pita and melt cheese. Dress with 3 large Romaine lettuce leaves (3), half of a fresh plum tomato, sliced (6), ¼ cup **sliced avocado** (96), and 2 Tbsp sliced onions (6).

Total Calories = 401

Southwest Veggie Burger: 1 Food For Life® Ezekiel 4:9® Sprouted Burger Bun (150) filled with 1 Gardenburger® Black Bean Chipotle Veggie Burger, microwaved (80), topped with ¼ cup **sliced avocado** (96), 2 Tbsp sliced onions (6), 1 sliced jalapeño (4), and 1 Tbsp salsa (10); 1 medium kiwi, sliced (46)

Total Calories = 392

Spaghetti & Meatballs: ¼ cup cooked whole wheat spaghetti (105), tossed with 1 Tbsp **extra virgin olive oil** (119), and topped with ½ cup Newman's Own® Marinara Pasta Sauce (60) and 6 Gardenburger® Mama Mia Veggie Meatballs, mirowaved (110)

Total Calories = 394

Spinach Black Bean Wrap: 1 Thomas'® Whole Wheat Sahara Wrap (170) filled with one Gardenburger® Black Bean Chipotle Veggie Burger, microwaved and chopped (80), topped with ½ cup fresh baby spinach leaves (3), 2 Tbsp chopped scallions (4), and ¼ cup **sliced avocado** (96)

Total Calories = 353

Tuna Pita: Half of a Thomas'® Multigrain Pita (70) filled with 2 ounces chunk light tuna in water (80), 2 diced sundried tomatoes jarred in extra virgin olive oil (20), 2 Tbsp chopped **walnuts** (185), and 1 Tbsp crumbled feta cheese (40)

Total Calories = 395

Tuna Salad: 2 cups organic mixed baby greens (15) tossed with 2 Tbsp Newman's Own® Light Balsamic Vinaigrette (45), topped with 2 oz chunk light water-packed tuna (80), 2 Tbsp **walnuts** (185), and 1 oz crumbled feta cheese (80)

Total Calories = 405

Turkey Cranberry Pita: 1 Thomas'® 100% Whole Wheat English Muffin (120) spread with 1 Laughing Cow® Light Garlic & Herb Wedge (35), filled with 2 oz Applegate Farms® Antibiotic-free Honey Maple Turkey (50), 1 Tbsp dried cranberries (45), and 2 Tbsp **walnuts** (185)

Total Calories = 435

Waldorf Pita: 1 Thomas'® Multigrain Pita (140) spread with 1 wedge Laughing Cow® Light Swiss Original (35), and filled with ¼ cup chopped celery (5), half of a medium apple, sliced (40), 2 Tbsp **walnuts** (185), and 3 large Romaine lettuce leaves (3)

Total Calories = 408

NOTES FROM OUR NUTRITIONIST

"Take Lunch, and That's an Order!"

A recent survey found that a whopping 74 percent of American office workers eat lunch at their desks. Eating while working can cause you to eat too fast, lose track of how much you've eaten, and distract you from the taste and enjoyment of your meal. Follow these lunchtime rules to help make your midday meal a priority:

- Set your cell phone or computer alarm to remind you to stop and eat. When it goes off, don't hit the snooze or dismiss it. You can pick up where you left off after your meal feeling reenergized.

- Commit to eating lunch with a co-worker. When you know a friend is waiting for you, you won't talk yourself into staying at your desk.

- Use real dishes and silverware. In Europe (where the average lunchtime is 50 percent longer but waistlines are smaller), people in France, Greece, Italy, Portugal, Spain, and other countries rely on this tradition to make each meal feel special. Store a set in your office kitchen—washing them will tack just a few seconds onto your meal.

- If you really have to eat at your desk, try not to work while you eat. Take a few deep breaths, and savor every bite—even if it's only for ten minutes.

—Cynthia

Dinner

Don't hesitate to whip up additional portions of these dinners for your family. Our testers raved and were so thankful that these options pleased husbands, kids, and teens alike! MUFAs are in boldface.

California Turkey Salad: 2 cups organic mixed baby greens (15) tossed with 2 Tbsp Newman's Own® Light Balsamic Vinaigrette (45) and topped with 3 oz browned all-breast-meat ground turkey (130), 2 Tbsp crumbled gorgonzola (50), and 2 Tbsp **walnuts** (185)

Total Calories = 425

Cheesy Veggie Pasta: ¼ cup fresh chopped red bell peppers (10), ½ cup broccoli florets (20), and 2 Tbsp sliced onions (6) sautéed in 1 Tbsp **extra virgin olive oil** (119) tossed with ¼ cup nonfat ricotta cheese (50), 2 Tbsp Organic Valley® Shredded Italian Four-Cheese Blend (45), and ¼ cup cooked whole wheat penne (105)

Total Calories = 355

Chicago-Style Hot Dog: 1 Lightlife® Jumbo Smart Dog (45) browned in skillet in 1 Tbsp **peanut oil** (119), on one Food For Life® Ezekiel 4:9® Sprouted Hot Dog Bun (170) dressed with 1 Tbsp mustard (0), 2 Tbsp sliced onions (6), 2 Tbsp sweet relish (30), half of a fresh plum tomato, diced (6), and a dash of celery seed

Total Calories = 376

Chicken Caesar: Chill 3 oz organic pre-cooked chicken breast (90) (optional: sear on grill). Toss 2 cups organic mixed baby greens (15) with mixture of 1 Tbsp **olive oil** (119) and 1 Tbsp Newman's Own® Lighten Up Caesar dressing (35). Top with chicken, 1 oz Asiago cheese (103), and 1 Ryvita® Dark Rye Crispbread cracker (35).

Total Calories = 397

Chicken Caprese: 2 oz organic grilled chicken breast (60) served with ½ cup steamed wild rice (150) and a tomato mozzarella salad made with 1 plum tomato, sliced (12), 1 oz sliced Polly-O® Part-Skim Mozzarella (70), and 2 fresh basil leaves (0) drizzled with 1 Tbsp **olive oil** (124) and 1 Tbsp balsamic vinegar (5) and dusted with cracked black pepper

Total Calories = 421

Edamame Salad: 2 cups organic mixed baby greens (15) tossed with 2 Tbsp Annie's Naturals® Goddess Dressing (90), topped with ⅔ cup Cascadian Farm® Organic Edamame, thawed (120), ¼ cup canned mandarin oranges, drained (40), and 2 Tbsp **almonds** (164)

Total Calories = 429

Edamame Wild Rice Salad: Chill ¼ cup cooked wild rice (75), and toss with ⅓ cup Cascadian Farm® Organic Edamame, thawed (60), 1 cup Cascadian Farm® Organic Chinese Stir-Fry vegetables, thawed (25), 2 Tbsp Annie's Naturals® Goddess Dressing (90), and 2 Tbsp **cashews** (163).

Total Calories = 413

Grilled Chicken Salad: 2 cups organic mixed baby greens (15) tossed with 2 Tbsp balsamic vinegar (10) and 1 Tbsp **extra virgin olive oil** (119) and topped with 3 oz organic grilled chicken breast (90), ½ cup broccoli florets (20), ¾ cup shredded carrots (38), ¼ cup sliced red onion (23), ¾ cup Cascadian Farm® Organic Sweet Corn, thawed (70), and sprinkle with fresh cracked black pepper

Total Calories = 385

Grilled Pork Salad: 3 oz pork tenderloin, grilled (115), served on a bed of 2 cups organic mixed baby greens (15) tossed with ½ cup drained pineapple tidbits (60), ¼ cup fresh chopped red bell peppers (10), ¼ cup crumbled feta (80), 2 Tbsp balsamic vinegar (10), and 1 Tbsp **extra virgin olive oil** (119)

Total Calories = 409

Mexicali Salad: 2 cups organic mixed baby greens (15) topped with ½ cup Amy's® Organic Refried Beans with Green Chiles (130), ¾ cup Cascadian Farm® Organic Sweet Corn, thawed (70), ¼ cup sliced red onion (23), ¼ cup salsa (40), and ¼ cup **sliced avocado** (96)

Total Calories = 374

Pepperoni Pizza: 1 flat Thomas'® Multigrain Pita (140) brushed on one side with 1 Tbsp **extra virgin olive oil** (119), and topped with ¼ cup Newman's Own® Marinara Pasta Sauce (30), 13 Lightlife® Smart Deli Pepperoni Slices (40), and 2 Tbsp Organic Valley® Shredded Italian Four-Cheese Blend (45); warm under broiler or in toaster oven to heat through

Total Calories = 374

Pineapple-Ham Pizza: 1 flat Thomas'® Multigrain Pita (140) brushed on one side with 1 Tbsp **extra virgin olive oil** (119) and topped with ¼ cup Newman's Own® Marinara Pasta Sauce (30), ¼ cup drained pineapple tidbits (30), ¼ cup fresh chopped red bell peppers (10), 2 oz Applegate Farms® uncured Black Forest ham, chopped (50), and 2 Tbsp crumbled gorgonzola (50); warm under broiler or in toaster oven to heat through

Total Calories = 429

Pork with Szechuan Vegetables: 2 cups Cascadian Farm® Organic Chinese Stir-Fry vegetables (50) sautéed in 1 Tbsp **canola oil** (124) flavored with ground szechuan peppercorns, served with 3 oz pork tenderloin, sliced (115), and ½ cup cooked Uncle Ben's® Ready Brown Rice (110)

Total Calories = 399

Ricotta Calzone: ¼ cup nonfat ricotta cheese (50) mixed with 2 sundried tomatoes jarred in olive oil, diced (20), 1 Tbsp **extra virgin olive oil** (119), 1 tsp minced garlic (10), and 4 fresh basil leaves, sliced (0). Stuff mixture into 1 Thomas'® Multigrain Pita (140). Warm under broiler until pita is golden and cheeses are bubbly. Serve with ½ cup Newman's Own® Marinara Pasta Sauce (60) for dipping.

Total Calories = 399

Salmon Pistachio Lettuce Wraps: 4 large Romaine lettuce leaves (4) filled evenly with 2 Tbsp dill hummus (50), ½ cup canned Alaskan salmon (180), half of a fresh plum tomato, diced (6), ¼ cup diced cucumber (5), and 2 Tbsp **pistachios** (161)

Total Calories = 406

Salmon Sandwich: 2 slices Food For Life® Ezekiel 4:9® Sesame Sprouted Bread (160) spread with 2 Tbsp **black olive tapenade** (88), ½ cup canned Alaskan salmon (180), half of a fresh plum tomato, diced (6) and 2 large Romaine lettuce leaves (2)

Total Calories = 436

Salmon Steak Almondine: 3 oz grilled wild Alaskan salmon (160) served with 1.5 cups frozen Cascadian Farm® Organic Cut Green Beans, steamed or microwaved (60) dressed with freshly ground white pepper and 2 Tbsp **sliced almonds** (164)

Total Calories = 384

Savory Turkey Pasta: ½ cup broccoli florets (20) and 1 cup plum tomato, sliced (30) sautéed in 1 Tbsp **extra virgin olive oil** (119), tossed with 4 fresh basil leaves, sliced (0), 3 oz browned all-breast-meat ground turkey (130), and ¼ cup cooked whole wheat penne (105)

Total Calories = 404

Sesame Ginger Shrimp Wrap: 1 Thomas'® Whole Wheat Sahara wrap (170) filled with 2 oz broiled medium shrimp (60), ¼ cup fresh snow peas (10), ¼ cup chopped celery (5), and 2 Tbsp **cashews** (163) drizzled with 1 Tbsp Newman's Own® Lighten Up Low Fat Sesame Ginger Dressing (18)

Total Calories = 426

Shrimp and Snow Pea Sesame Pasta: Chill 2 oz medium broiled shrimp (60) and ¼ cup cooked whole wheat spirals (105) and toss with 1 Tbsp **sesame oil** (120), ¼ cup fresh snow peas (10), 2 Tbsp chopped scallions (4), and ¼ cup chopped celery (5), and sprinkle with 1 Tbsp whole black sesame seeds (50).

Total Calories = 354

Slaw Dog: 1 Lightlife® Jumbo Smart Dog (45) browned in skillet in 1 Tbsp **peanut oil** (119), on one Food For Life® Ezekiel 4:9® Sprouted Hot Dog Bun (170) dressed with 1 Tbsp mustard (0), and half of a 12-ounce bag of Mann's® Broccoli Coleslaw mix (50) tossed with 2 Tbsp Newman's Own® Light Balsamic Vinaigrette (45)

Total Calories = 429

Spicy Shrimp: 3 oz medium shrimp, (90), brushed with 1 Tbsp China Blue® Spicy Chili Bean Glaze (40) and grilled, served with ½ cup steamed wild rice (150) and 1 cup fresh asparagus (30) sautéed in 1 Tbsp **canola oil** (124), 1 tsp minced garlic jarred in water (10), 1 Tbsp fresh chopped parsley (0), and freshly ground black pepper

Total Calories = 444

Spinach Burrito: 1 Thomas'® Whole Wheat Sahara wrap (170) filled with ½ cup fresh spinach (3), 1 tsp minced garlic (10), and ¼ cup sliced red onion (12) sautéed in 1 Tbsp **olive oil** (119), topped with 1 oz Asiago Fresco cheese (103)

Total Calories = 417

Szechuan Chicken: 2 cups frozen Cascadian Farm® Organic Chinese Stir-Fry vegetables (50) sautéed in 1 Tbsp **canola oil** (124) flavored with ground szechuan peppercorns, served with 3 oz organic grilled chicken breast (90) and ½ cup cooked Uncle Ben's® Ready Brown Rice (110)

Total Calories = 374

Turkey Quesadilla: Spread 1 Laughing Cow® Light Garlic & Herb Wedge (35) onto 1 Thomas'® Whole Wheat Sahara wrap (170). On half of wrap, place 2 oz Applegate Farms® Antibiotic-free Honey Maple Turkey (50), ¼ cup baby spinach leaves (1), 2 Tbsp crumbled feta (40), and 10 sliced **large black olives** (50). Fold over and heat in toaster oven or a nonstick pan over medium heat.

Total Calories = 346

Turkey Sauté: ½ cup fresh chopped red bell pepper (20) and ¼ cup sliced red onion (23) sautéed in 1 Tbsp **olive oil** (119), tossed with 2 Tbsp chopped scallions (4), 4 fresh basil leaves, sliced (0), and 3 oz browned all-breast-meat ground turkey (130), served with 3 oz (⅕ of bag) Alexia® Oven Fries with Olive Oil, Rosemary & Garlic, cooked under broiler or in toaster oven (120)

Total Calories = 416

Turkey Tacos: Sauté ¼ cup chopped red bell pepper (10) and 2 Tbsp sliced red onion (12) in 1 Tbsp **olive oil** (119). Brown 3 oz all-breast-meat ground turkey (130). Fill three 6-inch corn tortillas (135) evenly with turkey, then add pepper mixture and sprinkle with 2 Tbsp chopped scallions (4) and ¼ cup shredded carrots (14).

Total Calories = 424

Wild Salmon Cashew Salad: 2 cups organic mixed baby greens (15) tossed with 2 Tbsp Newman's Own® Lighten Up Low Fat Sesame Ginger Dressing (35) and topped with 3 oz grilled wild Alaskan salmon (160) and 2 Tbsp **cashews** (163)

Total Calories = 373

NOTES FROM OUR NUTRITIONIST

"The Cure for After-Work Munchies"

Many of the women I've counseled who work away from home eat lunch between noon and 1 p.m., but don't even start making dinner until well after 6 p.m. That means their hunger signals are in high gear before they even set foot in the kitchen—a perfect recipe for munching on pre-dinner snacks like crackers, chips, or cheese, or nibbling on meal ingredients while cooking. The best fix is to plan your Snack Pack in between lunch and dinner, around 3 or 4 p.m. The MUFA from your Snack Pack will help you stay full and satisfied, so you'll still feel energized (and even-tempered) when you start cooking. And because you won't be so ravenous, you won't rush through your meal prep.

—Cynthia

Flat Belly Ready-Made Meals

Pressed for time? Choose any of these options as a meal and you're good to go!

Meal Replacement Bars

CHOOSE 1 OF THE FOLLOWING MEAL REPLACEMENT BARS	CALORIES	ADD YOUR MUFA
● Clif® Black Cherry Almond Bar	250	
● Clif® Crunchy Peanut Butter Bar	250	
● Odwalla® Chocolate Chip Peanut bar	250	
● Clif® Chocolate Brownie bar	240	
Odwalla® Banana Nut bar	240	
● Nature's Path® Optimum® Pomegran Cherry energy bar	230	
● Larabar® Chocolate Coconut	220	
● Larabar® Banana Cookie	220	
● Larabar® Ginger Snap	220	2 Tbsp of (choose 1):
● Larabar® Apple Pie	210	Almonds (164)
● Larabar® Cinnamon Roll	210	Cashews (163)
● Nature's Path® Optimum® Blueberry Flax & Soy energy bar	200	Peanuts (166) Pistachios (161)
● Larabar® Pecan Pie	200	Pumpkin seeds (148)
● Nature's Path® Optimum® Cranberry Zen energy bar	200	
● Larabar® Cherry Pie	190	
● Luna® Chai Tea bar	180	
● Luna® Chocolate Pecan Pie bar	180	
● Luna® Lemon Zest bar	180	
● Luna® Nutz Over Chocolate™ bar	180	
● Luna® Peanut Butter Cookie bar	180	
● Luna® S'mores bar	180	

Frozen Meals

CHOOSE 1 OF THE FOLLOWING MEALS	CALORIES	ADD YOUR MUFA
● Amy's® Chili & Cornbread Dinner	340	10 large green or black olives (or 5 of each) (50)
● Kashi® Black Bean Mango	340	
● Amy's® Black Bean Enchilada Dinner	330	
● Kashi® Lemon Rosemary Chicken	330	
● Amy's® Indian Mattar Paneer	320	
● Kashi® Sweet & Sour Chicken	320	
● Seeds of Change® Moroccan Lentil Tagine	320	
● Amy's® Indian Vegetable Korma	300	
● Seeds of Change® Hanalei Vegetarian Chicken Teriyaki	300	
● Amy's® Organic Brown Rice, Black-Eyed Peas & Veggies Bowl	290	
● Amy's® Organic Teriyaki Bowl	280	
● Amy's® Veggie Loaf Dinner	280	
● Kashi® Chicken Pasta Pomodoro	280	
● Seeds of Change® Lasagna Calabrese with Eggplant and Portobello Mushrooms	270	
● Amy's® Indian Mattar Tofu	260	2 Tbsp pumpkin seeds (148)
● Kashi® Lime Cilantro Shrimp	250	
● Gardenburger® Black Bean Chipotle Wrap	240	
● Gardenburger® Margherita Pizza Wrap	240	
● Kashi® Southwest Style Chicken	240	
● Cedarlane™ Three Layer Enchilada Pie	215	2 Tbsp Brazil nuts (186)
● Cedarlane™ Low Fat Garden Vegetable Lasagna	180	

Fast Food

MENU ITEM (S)	CALORIES	ADD YOUR MUFA
● Baja Fresh® Baja Ensalada with Charbroiled Chicken with Salsa	325	10 large green or black olives (or 5 of each) (50)
● Jack in the Box® Asian Grilled Chicken Salad with Roasted Slivered Almonds and Low-Fat Balsamic Dressing	310	
● Pizza Hut® Fit n' Delicious™ Pizza (two slices) with Green pepper, Red Onion & Diced Tomato (12")	300	
● Fazoli's® Chicken and Fruit Salad with Fat-Free Honey Mustard	280	
● Arby's® Junior Roast Beef Sandwich	273	
● Chick-fil-A® Chargrilled Chicken Sandwich	270	
● Jamba Juice® Berry Fulfilling® smoothie (24 oz)	260	2 Tbsp of pumpkin seeds (148)
● Boston Market® roasted turkey breast (180) with poultry gravy (15) and steamed vegetables (60)	255	
● Taco Bell® Chicken Enchirito® (Fresco Style)	250	
● Wendy's® Small Chili	220	2 Tbsp pistachios (161)
● Domino's® Grilled Chicken Caesar with Light Italian Dressing	220	2 Tbsp almonds (164)
● Panera® Low-Fat Vegetarian Garden Vegetable Soup (8 oz) with a Whole Grain Loaf	220	
● McDonald's® Asian Salad with Grilled Chicken and Newman's Own® Low-Fat Sesame Ginger Dressing	180	
● Au Bon Pain® Jamaican Black Bean Soup (medium)	180	
● Taco Bell® Ranchero Chicken Soft Taco (Fresco Style)	170	2 Tbsp peanuts (166)
● Subway® Oven Roasted Chicken Breast Salad with Fat Free Italian Dressing and Roasted Chicken Noodle Soup	175 / 80	2 Tbsp pumpkin seeds (148)
● Panda Express® String Bean Chicken Breast with Mixed Vegetables	160 / 90	

Questions Anyone?

Cynthia answers some of your most common and pressing queries.

Q: *Can I swap out ingredients in a meal?*

A: Yes and no. You should not move items from one meal to another—that is, you can't take your MUFA from breakfast and add it to lunch. But you *can* swap out foods within a meal, as long as:

* they're within the same food group, such as trading tomatoes for red peppers or turkey for chicken; and

* the food you added provides about the same number of calories as the food you took out. As I noted on page 119, the calories for each ingredient appear in parentheses.

Q: *I see that the plan includes name brand foods. Do I have to buy these exact brands?*

A: I selected these particular brands because of their taste, quality, availability, and, most importantly, nutritional value. As a registered dietitian and *Prevention's* "Grocery Guru" columnist, I've found that the nutritional quality of foods in certain categories varies widely. So I scoured the supermarket aisles, read countless labels, and hand-picked the high-quality brands that meet my tough nutritional standards. I am also sure that including these foods will provide exactly the right number of calories because I know their precise calorie level per serving. So, yes, I encourage you to use these brands. However, if you can't or prefer not to, please choose a comparable food with as close to exactly the same calorie level.

Q: *Why are some of the foods on the diet organic but not all?*

A: Studies have found that organically grown foods do contain higher levels of anti-aging, immune-boosting, disease-fighting nutrients. Therefore, eating at least some organic foods can up your diet's overall nutritional "bang-for-the-buck." Many people also believe that organic foods taste better, and if your meals are more flavorful and satisfying, you may be less tempted to give into the urge to sneak a pint of Ben & Jerry's into your cart at the market. However, organic foods can be more expensive, and convenience is key.

(continued on page 142)

READ A FLAT BELLY
SUCCESS STORY

Julie Plavsic
Age: 42
Pounds lost: 6 in 32 days
All-over inches lost: 7.5

"I had a baby a couple of years ago and since then— until now, anyway—I've been struggling with ten stubborn pounds. I was on the lower end of what I needed to lose, but I just couldn't get the scale to budge. I was eating healthy. Exercising. Nothing seemed to be working. Of course, I have to confess, I didn't have the most perfect eating habits at the time."

Julie admits to many of the behaviors that lead to a dieter's downfall. She was grazing on "stuff" all day long, she says. And she wasn't always honest with herself about what and how much she was eating. "Like pasta. I was having what I thought was a small serving of pasta, but according to the *Flat Belly Diet*, I was actually having a double or a triple portion. Who really measures? It looked like a small portion, so I told myself it was fine."

Other diets? Julie had tried them all. She couldn't recall the number of times

before

after

she was on the famous low-carb diet, but it was at least a few. She found it "torture" and worse, felt it wasn't sustainable. When she heard about the *Flat Belly Diet*, she thought it just might work. "I knew I needed the structure of a diet that would tell me what to do, so I figured I'd check it out."

At first, looking at 1,600 calories a day, she didn't think she could do it. But it wasn't hard, she claims, because the food is so filling. The MUFAs, the core of it, amazed her. She tried dozens of things on the menu the first couple of weeks, but in the end, she needed to simplify. Julie, who works as an immigration lawyer and with her job and small baby, needed to ration her time. She needed meals that she could create quickly. "So I ended up having the same thing every morning—peanut butter on toast—which I love. And after that, I was full until lunch. No more snacking all morning."

What was hard for her, she claims, was changing her thinking in so many ways. "I knew that the diet required us to eat things like olives and olive oil. And even though I knew that the calories were not that bad, it was hard, at first, for me to believe it that you can fight fat by eating fat. Or that fat has to do with other things as well. I had to get over all those years of denying myself those high-fat foods. It was a leap of faith."

NOW

It was a leap she's glad she took. "I learned so much from this diet," she says. "First of all, I learned that belly fat can be more dangerous than the other kinds of fat, and so with this diet, I'm making my body healthier in addition to making it thinner. And that's good, because I'm much more inclined to stick to a diet that I know is doing something healthy for my body. I also learned that what the scale says is so much less important than how you feel. I wanted to get to 130, but I'm happy with how I look and how my clothes fit at 133."

Julie doesn't consider what she's doing a "diet," per se. For her, it's more a new way of looking at food, of making choices and using calories wisely, a way of portioning out what you need to put in each meal throughout the day. "I'm thinking about all the overweight friends I have," she says. "I'm so excited by this diet, I can't *wait* to get them to try it!"

Organic baby carrots are essentially ready-to-eat, and if they taste better and provide more nutrition, they may be well worth the 50 cents extra they cost compared to conventionally grown baby carrots. So, if possible, do try to use the name brand organic items I've selected. If you can't or don't want to, no big deal. Just be sure to choose a similar item with the same (or as close as possible) calorie level.

Q. *If I eat a pound of food, will I gain a pound of weight?*

A. A half-gallon of water weighs 4 pounds, but if you drink a half-gallon of water, you won't gain 4 pounds of fat. You will, however, temporarily weigh 4 pounds more on the scale—that is, until your kidneys eliminate that water. That's because when you step on that scale, you are weighing anything that has weight to it—the water you just drank, the undigested food you ate a few hours ago, the waste from the food you ate yesterday that hasn't worked its way all the way through your GI tract yet, your muscle, skeleton, and body fat, and the clothes you're wearing (if any).

Most of the weight fluctuations we see on a scale have to do with our fluid status, because that's the variable that changes the most from hour to hour and day to day. If you're retaining water, you could easily weigh 5 pounds more, and if you're dehydrated (maybe from being sick), you could weigh 5 pounds less. Changes in actual body fat, however, happen much slower and are controlled solely by calories. It takes an excess of 3,500 calories (that means above and beyond the calories you burn) to create 1 pound of body fat. If you ate 700 calories more than your body could burn in 1 day, you'd gain $\frac{1}{5}$ of a pound. Do that 5 days in a row starting on a Monday, and by the end of the workweek, you've accumulated 1 pound of fat. (By the way, a pound of fat is nothing to sneeze at; it's equal to 4 sticks of butter!). So, while that number staring back at you seems to jump up and down like a yo-yo, you can see that it really takes several days in a row of overeating to even gain 1 pound of actual body fat. The scale is much less fickle when it comes to fat than water!

Create Your Own Favorite Menu

Members of **www.flatbellydiet.com** automatically receive a daily or weekly menu plan, complete with a printable shopping list. If any one of these meals—or even individual foods—simply doesn't do it for you, swap it for another of equal calories and MUFA content. (The system pre-programs a list of choices so you don't have to do any tricky math!) Plus, the interactive Food Log allows you to designate certain items as "favorites" so they'll quickly pop up when you're searching for another replacement. Hey, I wish we could cook the meals for you, but our tech team hasn't quite figured that out yet . . . !

www.flatbellydiet.com

The Four-Week Plan— The Flat Belly Diet Recipes

I have a confession to make. I'm not a big cook. I have my specialties (well, specialty: an hors d'oeuvre of mini pumpernickel slices spread with a melted cheddar, olive and curry mixture) that I rely on whenever I have company, but for the most part, my husband's the chef in the house. He's also, bless his heart, the one who does most of the grocery shopping. I'm good at saying what I like (helpfully encouraging him to make things that are fresh, healthy, vegetable-filled, and filling) and what would be better served when I'm away on a business trip.

Now why, you're probably wondering, would Liz start off the recipe chapter with a confession like that? Because if I see a recipe that has 100 ingredients and takes a day to prepare, my eyes glaze over and I start thinking about ordering a pizza. So I vowed that any recipe chapter in a book of mine needed to be filled with dishes I could envision myself making.

To that end, the recipes you'll find here are sufficiently gourmet to make your mouth water and get your creative chef juices flowing. But they're also extremely simple. Take the Pumpkin Spiced Oatmeal on page 154. *It takes 2 minutes! (My kinda recipe, that!)* Or the Sweet and Sour Shrimp on page 206—a mere 15 minutes start to finish. And believe me, the flavors will astound you.

But what makes these recipes extraordinary is not how easy or fast they are to prepare, but how well they fit into the Flat Belly Diet. Each recipe serving contains a MUFA, for starters. You can spot them in the ingredients lists by looking for the shaded line and star. As you know, MUFAs are the only foods that can specifically help reduce belly fat. In addition, beside each recipe is a very important box titled "Make It a Flat Belly Diet Meal." This box tells you what to add to one serving of that recipe to turn it into a Flat Belly Diet meal that you can slot right into your menu plan. In other words, let's say you decide to start your day with a serving of the delicious Apple Pancakes on page 152. Your MUFA is included. But remember that every meal on the Flat Belly Diet should equal roughly 400 calories. When you sit down to your delicious 209-calorie Apple Pancake breakfast, you should also add 1 cup of skim milk (80 calories) and 3 slices of turkey bacon (90 calories) to round out the meal and raise it to the appropriate calorie level healthfully.

Confused? Don't be. All you have to do is follow the instructions in the "Make It a Flat Belly Diet Meal" boxes at the end of each recipe and you'll be assured of staying within the Flat Belly Diet rules, no matter which recipes you choose to try. Now let's get cookin'.

BREAKFASTS pp. 151–157

Frittata with Smoked Salmon and Scallions

Apple Pancakes

Nutty Fruit Muffins

Pumpkin Spiced Oatmeal

Southwestern Double-Corn & Pecan Muffins

Fluted Egg Cups

Fiesta Cornmeal Pudding

SANDWICHES pp. 158–160

Grilled Portobello and Roasted Pepper Burgers

Wasabi Salmon Sandwiches

Tuna Bruschetta

SOUPS pp. 161–168

Fresh Pea Soup with Mint

Asian Soup with Shrimp Dumplings

Mexican Chicken Soup

Slow Cooker Chili

Black Bean Chili

Hearty Country Vegetable Soup

Turnip and Carrot Soup with Parmesan

Chilled Strawberry Soup

SALADS pp. 169–182

Cucumber and Melon Salad with Watercress, Herbs, and Feta

Crab Salad with Avocado and Pomelo

Curried Barley and Shrimp Salad

Warm Quinoa Salad

Italian Shrimp and Pasta Salad

Turkey-Avocado Cobb Salad

Soba Noodle Salad with Snow Peas

Spinach Salad

Herb and Mesclun Salad with Grilled Shrimp

Curried Potato Salad

Bitter Greens with Hot Vinaigrette Dressing

Moroccan Carrot Salad with Toasted Cumin

Spinach Salad with Radishes and Walnuts

Strawberry and Red Onion Salad

POULTRY pp. 183–198

Crisp Romaine Salad with Chicken and Mango

Greek Lemon Chicken

Spinach-Stuffed Chicken Roulade

Chicken with Citrus-Avocado Salsa

Grilled Ginger-Soy Chicken

Grilled Oregano Chicken

Lime-Marinated Chicken with Salsa

Grape-ful Chicken

Almond-Encrusted Chicken Breast

Chicken with Orange Almond Topping

Chicken with Banana Chutney Topping

Chicken with Raspberry Topping

Chicken with Honey Mustard and Pecan Topping

Zesty Chicken Fiesta

Tuscan Chicken with Beans

Hearty Brussels Sprouts with Sausage

SEAFOOD pp. 199–210

Steamed Salmon with Snow Peas

Fish with Summer Squash

Roasted Fish with Artichokes

Grilled Salmon Steak

Lemony Stuffed Sole

Scallop Ceviche

Chai Scallops with Bok Choy

Sweet and Sour Shrimp

Sizzled Shrimp with Heirloom Tomatoes

Sesame Seared Scallops

Thai Sweet-Hot Shrimp

Seared Wild Salmon with Mango Salsa

MEAT pp. 211–215

Dijon Pork Chops with Cabbage

Mexican Pork Tenderloin

Stir-Fried Rice with Asian Vegetables and Beef

Vietnamese Beef Salad

Basic Balsamic Flank Steak

VEGETARIAN pp. 216–222

Broccoli and Tofu Stir-Fry with Toasted Almonds

Quick Chicks

Zucchini Rotini

Stewed Vegetables

Stir-Fried Broccoli and Mushrooms with Tofu

Spaghetti Squash Casserole

Soybeans with Sesame and Scallions

SIDE DISHES pp. 223–232

Beet and Goat Cheese Salad

Balsamic Roasted Carrots

Mini Sweet Potato Casseroles

Summer Squash Sauté

Carrot-Walnut Salad

Sugar Snap Pea and Fennel Salad with Apple Cider Vinaigrette

Wild Rice, Almond, and Cranberry Dressing

Guilt-Free Fries

Stir-Fried Asparagus with Ginger, Sesame, and Soy

Tuscan White Bean Spread

DESSERTS pp. 233–238

Plum and Nectarine Trifle

Chocolate Strawberries

Pumpkin-Maple Cheesecake

Oatmeal Cookies with Cranberries and Chocolate Chips

Chocolate Pudding with Bananas and Graham Crackers

Citrus Ricotta Cannoli

Parentheses Basics

The numbers in parentheses in the "Make It a Flat Belly Diet Meal" boxes correspond to the calorie count of each ingredient. They will help you become familiar with the calorie levels of various ingredients and also aid you in customizing your plan.

Frittata with Smoked Salmon and Scallions

Preparation time: 10 minutes | Cooking time: 15 minutes

2 teaspoons extra virgin olive oil

6 scallions (whites and 2" of green), trimmed and coarsely chopped

6 egg whites

4 eggs

1½ teaspoons chopped fresh tarragon or ½ teaspoon dried

¼ cup cold water

½ teaspoon salt

Freshly ground black pepper

2 ounces thinly sliced smoked salmon, cut into ½"-wide pieces

¾ cup black olive tapenade

1. Preheat the oven to 350°F. Heat a heavy 8" ovenproof skillet over medium heat for 1 minute. Add the olive oil and scallions and sauté, stirring, or until soft.

2. In a medium bowl, whisk together the egg whites, eggs, tarragon, water, and salt. Season with the black pepper. Pour the mixture into the pan and lay salmon pieces on top. Cook, stirring periodically, for about 2 minutes or until partially set.

3. Transfer to the oven and roast for about 6 to 8 minutes, or until firm, golden, and puffed. Remove. Use a spatula to release frittata from the pan. Gently slide the frittata onto a warm serving platter. Spread 2 tablespoons of the tapenade on each plate, and place a slice of frittata on top.

Makes 6 servings

Per serving: 190 calories, 10 g protein, 2 g carbohydrates, 15 g fat, 2.5 g saturated fat, 143 mg cholesterol, 537 mg sodium, 0 g fiber

Make It a Flat Belly Diet Meal

Serve with ½ cup frozen dark cherries, thawed (45) mixed into 1 cup nonfat plain Greek yogurt (112) topped with 2 tablespoons toasted oats (37) Total calories: 384

Apple Pancakes

Preparation time: 20 minutes | Cooking time: 4 minutes

²/₃ cup whole wheat flour

²/₃ cup unbleached all-purpose flour

¹/₃ cup cornmeal

1 tablespoon baking powder

1 teaspoon ground ginger

¹/₂ teaspoon baking soda

2 cups nonfat plain yogurt

³/₄ cup fat-free egg substitute

2 tablespoons canola oil

1 apple, peeled, cored, and coarsely grated

1¹/₂ cups chopped pecans

1. In a large bowl, combine the flours, cornmeal, baking powder, ginger, baking soda, yogurt, egg substitute, and oil until combined.

2. Fold the grated apples into the batter.

3. Coat a large, nonstick skillet with nonstick cooking spray and heat over medium heat.

4. For each pancake, spoon 2 to 3 tablespoons (25 to 45 ml) of the batter into the skillet. Cook for 2 minutes or until bubbles appear on the surface and edges set. Flip to the other side.

5. Cook until lightly browned, about 2 minutes. Repeat with the remaining batter.

6. Top each serving with 2 tablespoons chopped pecans.

Makes 12 servings

Per serving: 209 calories, 6 g protein, 19 g carbohydrates, 13.5 g fat, 1 g saturated fat, 1 mg cholesterol, 208 mg sodium, 3 g fiber

Make It a Flat Belly Diet Meal

Serve with 1 cup skim milk (80) and 3 slices Applegate Farms® Organic Turkey Bacon (90)

Total calories: 379

Nutty Fruit Muffins

Preparation time: 10 minutes | Cooking time: 20 minutes

1¾ cups whole grain pastry flour
1½ teaspoons baking powder
1½ teaspoons ground cinnamon
½ teaspoon baking soda
¼ teaspoon salt
1 cup fat-free vanilla yogurt
½ cup brown sugar
1 egg
2 tablespoons canola oil
1 teaspoon vanilla extract
1½ cups chopped walnuts
½ cup crushed pineapple in juice, drained
⅓ cup currants or raisins
¼ cup grated carrots

1. Preheat the oven to 400°F.

2. In a large bowl, combine first five ingredients. In a medium bowl, combine the yogurt, brown sugar, egg, oil, and vanilla extract. Stir the yogurt mixture into the flour mixture just until blended. (Lumps are OK.) Fold in the walnuts, pineapple, currants or raisins, and carrots.

3. Divide the batter evenly among 12 muffin cups coated with nonstick cooking spray.

4. Bake for 20 minutes or until a toothpick inserted in the center of a muffin comes out clean.

5. Cool in pan on a wire rack for 5 minutes. Remove muffins from the pan to cool completely on the wire rack.

Makes 12 servings

Per serving: 242 calories, 6 g protein, 29 g carbohydrates, 12.5 g fat, 1 g saturated fat, 18 mg cholesterol, 177 mg sodium, 3 g fiber

Make It a Flat Belly Diet Meal
Serve with 1 cup nonfat plain Greek yogurt (112)
Total calories: 354

Pumpkin Spiced Oatmeal

Preparation and Cooking time: 2 minutes

- 1 cup water
- Pinch of salt
- ⅓ cup quick oats
- ¼ cup canned pure pumpkin
- ★ 2 tablespoons toasted chopped pecans
- ¼ teaspoon ground cinnamon
- 2 teaspoons brown sugar
- Pinch of freshly grated nutmeg
- Pinch of ground cloves

1. In a saucepan over high heat, bring the water to a boil. Add the salt and oats. Cook, stirring for 90 seconds.

2. Combine the remaining ingredients in a small bowl. Reduce the heat to low and stir in the pumpkin mixture.

Adjust spices to taste.

Makes 1 serving

Per serving: 272 calories, 6 g protein, 36 g carbohydrates, 13 g fat, 1 g saturated fat, 0 mg cholesterol, 305 mg sodium, 7 g fiber

Make It a Flat Belly Diet Meal
Serve with 1 cup skim milk (80)
Total calories: 352

Southwestern Double-Corn & Pecan Muffins

Preparation time: 5 minutes | Cooking time: 18 minutes

- 1 cup yellow cornmeal
- 1 cup whole grain pastry flour
- ¼ cup soy flour
- 2 teaspoons baking powder
- ¼ teaspoon ground cinnamon
- ⅛ teaspoon salt
- 1 egg
- 1 egg white
- ¾ cup skim milk
- ¼ cup canola oil
- 1½ cups frozen corn kernels
- ★ 1½ cups chopped pecans
- ½ cup golden raisins

1. Preheat the oven to 400°F

2. In a large bowl, combine the cornmeal, pastry flour, soy flour, baking powder, cinnamon, and salt.

3. In a small bowl, combine the egg, egg white, milk, oil, corn, pecans, and raisins. Add the egg mixture to the flour mixture and stir just until blended. (Lumps are OK.) Fold in corn kernels, pecans, and raisins. Divide the batter evenly among 12 muffin cups coated with nonstick cooking spray.

4. Bake for 18 minutes or until a toothpick inserted in the center of a muffin comes out clean. Cool in the pan on a wire rack for 5 minutes. Remove from the pan to cool completely on the wire rack.

Makes 12 servings

Per serving: 273 calories, 6 g protein, 27 g carbohydrates, 17.5 g fat, 2 g saturated fat, 19 mg cholesterol, 113 mg sodium, 4 g fiber

Make It a Flat Belly Diet Meal

Serve with 1 cup skim milk (80)

Total calories: 353

Fluted Egg Cups

Preparation time: 10 minutes | Cooking time: 5 minutes | Baking time:
20 minutes | Broiling time: 2 minutes

    6 large slices 100% whole-wheat bread
    2 tablespoons olive oil
  ⅓ cup chopped scallions
    1 tablespoon chopped fresh basil
    1 tablespoon chopped fresh Italian parsley
    8 egg whites, lightly beaten
  ⅓ cup (about 1½ ounces) shredded reduced fat Cheddar cheese
    1 tablespoon grated Parmesan cheese
  ½ teaspoon paprika
  1½ cups black olive tapenade

1. Preheat the oven to 350°F. With a rolling pin, slightly flatten the bread slices. Using a 3" round cookie cutter, cut 12 bread circles.

2. Coat a 12-cup mini-muffin pan with nonstick cooking spray. Line each cup with a bread round. Bake for 15 to 20 minutes, or until the edges are golden-brown.

3. Heat the oil in a large nonstick skillet over medium heat. Add the scallions, basil, and parsley; cook, stirring, for 1 to 2 minutes. Add the egg whites. Cook, stirring with a wooden spoon, for 1 to 2 minutes or until almost set. Fold in the cheese and cook until the eggs are set.

4. Preheat the broiler. Spoon 1 tablespoon of the egg mixture into each bread cup and top with the Parmesan and paprika. Broil 4" from the heat source for 1 to 2 minutes, or until hot and lightly browned. Serve each cup with 2 tablespoons of the tapenade.

Makes 12 servings

Per serving: 172 calories, 6 g protein, 6 g carbohydrates, 13 g fat, 2 g saturated fat, 3 mg cholesterol, 324 mg sodium, 1 g fiber

Make It a Flat Belly Diet Meal

Serve with ½ cup frozen dark cherries, thawed (45) mixed 1 cup nonfat Greek yogurt (112), and sprinkled with 2 tablespoons toasted oats (37)

Total calories: 366

Fiesta Cornmeal Pudding

Preparation time: 10 minutes | Cooking time: 20 minutes | Baking time: 30 minutes

2¼ cups water
½ teaspoon salt
¾ cup yellow cornmeal
1 tablespoon extra virgin olive oil
1 large red bell pepper, seeded and diced
4 scallions, chopped
2 large cloves garlic, minced
1½ cups chopped pecans, divided
1 box (10 ounces) frozen chopped spinach, thawed and squeezed dry
1 large egg white
¼ teaspoon hot pepper sauce
½ cup (2 ounces) shredded sharp Cheddar cheese

1. Preheat the oven to 350°F.

2. Coat a 9" baking dish with nonstick cooking spray.

3. In a large saucepan over high heat, bring the water to a boil. Add the salt. Reduce the heat to low. Whisk in the cornmeal in a slow, steady stream. Cover and cook, stirring frequently, for 10 minutes or until very thick.

4. Meanwhile, heat the oil in a nonstick skillet over medium heat. Add the bell pepper; cook, stirring, for 4 minutes. Add the scallions and garlic; cook, stirring, for 2 minutes or until the vegetables are tender. Add the bell pepper mixture, 1 cup of the pecans, spinach, egg white, and hot pepper sauce to the cornmeal. Stir to combine. Pour into the prepared baking dish. Sprinkle with the Cheddar.

5. Bake for 30 minutes or until firm, puffed, and golden. Top with remaining pecans.

Makes 6 servings

Per serving: 344 calories, 9 g protein, 21 g carbohydrates, 26 g fat, 3.5 g saturated fat, 7 mg cholesterol, 372 mg sodium, 4 g fiber

Make It a Flat Belly Diet Meal

Serve with 2 slices Applegate Farms® Organic Bacon (60)
Total calories: 404

Grilled Portobello and Roasted Pepper Burgers

Preparation time: 4 minutes | Cooking time: 6 minutes

- 4 small portobello mushroom caps (8 ounces total), stems removed
- 4 teaspoons balsamic vinegar
- 2 jarred, roasted red bell pepper halves
- 2 100% whole wheat buns
- 2 tablespoons prepared pesto
- 4 leaves frisée lettuce

1. Preheat a grill pan over medium heat.

2. Grill the mushrooms for 8 minutes, turning halfway during cooking and brushing with the vinegar. Warm the pepper halves and buns on the grill pan.

3. Place 2 mushrooms and 1 pepper slice on each bun bottom, adding 2 pieces of frisée to each. Drizzle with additional vinegar, if desired, cap with bun top.

Makes 2 servings

Per serving: 270 calories, 10 g protein, 37 g carbohydrates, 9.5 g fat, 2.5 g saturated fat, 5 mg cholesterol, 614 mg sodium, 5 g fiber

Make It a Flat Belly Diet Meal

Add a dessert: Mix ¼ cup nonfat ricotta cheese (50) with 1 teaspoon honey (21) and top with ½ cup pear slices (50)

Total calories: 391

Wasabi Salmon Sandwiches

Preparation time: 8 minutes

- ¼ cup fat-free mayonnaise
- ¼–½ teaspoon wasabi paste
- 2 cups (about 8 ounces) canned Alaskan wild salmon
- 8 thin slices 100% whole wheat bread, toasted
- 4 thin slices red onion
- 4 thin rings red bell pepper, seeded
- 1 cup sliced avocado
- ¼ cup sliced pickled ginger
- 1 cup arugula

1. In a small bowl, combine the mayonnaise and wasabi paste until smooth. Start with ¼ teaspoon of the paste and add more to suit your taste. Gently fold in the salmon.

2. Place 4 slices of the bread on a flat surface and top each with ½ cup of the salmon mixture, 1 onion slice separated into rings, 1 pepper ring, ¼ cup avocado, 1 tablespoon ginger, and ¼ cup arugula. Top with the remaining 4 slices of bread.

Makes 4 servings

Per serving: 243 calories, 12 g protein, 26 g carbohydrates, 10 g fat, 1.5 g saturated fat, 21 mg cholesterol, 355 mg sodium, 6 g fiber

Make It a Flat Belly Diet Meal

Serve with ⅔ cup frozen, thawed Cascadian Farm® Organic Edamame (120)
Total calories: 363

Tuna Bruschetta

Preparation time: 5 minutes

  1 can (6 ounces) reduced-sodium water-packed tuna, drained and flaked
  1 cup canned no-salt-added, diced tomatoes, drained
  ¼ cup (1 ounce) crumbled reduced-fat feta cheese
  ¼ cup black olive tapenade
  1 tablespoon lemon juice
  4 slices 100% whole wheat bread, toasted

1. In a bowl, combine the tuna, tomatoes, feta, and lemon juice.

2. Spread the tapenade over 2 slices of the toast and top each with half of the tuna mixture. Top with the remaining 2 slices of toast.

Makes 2 servings

Per serving: 391 calories, 35 g protein, 30 g carbohydrates, 14.5 fat, 2.5 g saturated fat, 43 mg cholesterol, 717 mg sodium, 6 g fiber

Fresh Pea Soup with Mint

Preparation time: 7 minutes | Cooking time: 15 minutes | Chilling time: 1 hour

- 1 tablespoon olive oil
- 2 scallions, green parts only, cut into 4" pieces
- 1 rib celery, trimmed and cut into 2" pieces
- ½ medium onion, finely chopped
- 3 cups low-sodium chicken or vegetable broth
- 4 cups peas, fresh, or frozen and thawed
- ¼ teaspoon salt
- ⅓ cup fresh mint leaves
- ½ cup nonfat plain Greek yogurt
- ⭐ ½ cup toasted pumpkin seeds

1. Heat the oil in large sauce pot over medium-high heat. Add the scallions, celery, and onion. Cook, stirring, for about 5 minutes, or until the vegetables are tender.

2. Add the broth and bring to a boil. Add the peas and salt. Simmer for 10 minutes.

3. Carefully transfer the mixture to the bowl of a food processor fitted with a metal blade, or into a blender (in batches, if necessary). Add the mint. Puree until smooth. Cover and chill for at least 1 hour.

4. Spoon the soup into 4 serving bowls. Dollop 2 tablespoons of yogurt in the center of each, and sprinkle with 2 tablespoons of pumpkin seeds.

Makes 4 servings

Per serving: 337 calories, 23 g protein, 29 g carbohydrates, 16.5 g fat, 3 g saturated fat, 4 mg cholesterol, 439 mg sodium, 8 g fiber

Make It a Flat Belly Diet Meal

Serve with 1 cup grapes (60)
Total calories: 397

Asian Soup with Shrimp Dumplings

Preparation time: 15 minutes | Cooking time: 15 minutes

   4 cloves garlic, smashed, divided
½" piece fresh ginger, peeled and smashed, divided
½ pound medium shrimp, peeled and deveined
¼ cup fresh cilantro
   2 teaspoons cornstarch
   2 tablespoons water
   1 tablespoon reduced-sodium soy sauce
½ teaspoon toasted sesame oil
   6 cups low-sodium chicken broth
   1 stalk lemongrass, cut in half and smashed
½ teaspoon red pepper flakes
   1 cup cooked kale
½ cup chopped, dry-roasted peanuts

1. In a food processor, mince half of the garlic and ginger. Add the shrimp and cilantro; pulse to combine. In a small bowl, whisk together the cornstarch and water until the cornstarch is dissolved. Add to the food processor along with the soy sauce and oil. Pulse to combine. Set aside.

2. In a large saucepan over high heat, bring to a boil the broth, lemongrass, red pepper flakes, and the remaining garlic and ginger. Reduce the heat to low and let simmer.

3. Meanwhile, moisten your clean hands and roll the shrimp mixture into 12 balls. Drop the shrimp dumplings one at a time into the simmering soup. Cook for 6 minutes or until opaque. Remove and discard the lemongrass. Divide the greens evenly among 4 serving bowls and ladle the soup and 3 dumplings on top of each. Sprinkle with 2 tablespoons of peanuts.

Makes 4 servings

Per serving: 252 calories, 24 g protein, 13 g carbohydrates, 13 g fat, 2 g saturated fat, 86 mg cholesterol, 335 mg sodium, 2 g fiber

Make It a Flat Belly Diet Meal

Serve with 1 cup red pepper slices (40) and ¼ cup hummus for dipping (100)
Total calories: 392

Mexican Chicken Soup

Preparation time: 4 minutes | Cooking time: 16 minutes

 5 cups low-sodium chicken broth
 5 white corn tortillas (6"), sliced into ¼" strips
 12 ounces boneless, skinless chicken breast, thinly sliced crosswise
 ½ canned chipotle chile pepper, sliced, or 2 tablespoons hot salsa
 ¾ cup halved grape tomatoes
 1 cup chopped avocado
 ¼ cup fresh cilantro leaves

1. In a large, heavy saucepan, bring the broth to a boil, covered over high heat.

2. Meanwhile, scatter the tortilla strips on a toaster oven tray. Toast, turning the strips occasionally, until golden-brown in spots, about 5 minutes. Remove the tray from toaster oven and set the tortilla strips aside.

3. When the broth boils, add the chicken, chile pepper, and tomatoes and return to a boil. Remove from the heat. Divide the tortilla strips, avocado, and cilantro leaves evenly among 4 bowls, mounding them in the center. Ladle the soup into bowls.

Makes 4 servings

Per serving: 282 calories, 29 g protein, 24 g carbohydrates, 9.5 g fat, 1.5 g saturated fat, 49 mg cholesterol, 153 mg sodium, 5 g fiber

Make It a Flat Belly Diet Meal

Serve with 2 cups baby greens (10) tossed with 2 tablespoons Newman's Own® Light Balsamic Vinaigrette (45) and 1½ cups of grapes (60)
Total calories: 397

Slow Cooker Chili

Preparation time: 10 minutes | Cooking time: 4 to 6 hours

- 1 can (28 ounces) salt-free whole tomatoes
- 1 medium green bell pepper, seeded and chopped
- 1 can (14 ounces) chili beans, rinsed and drained
- ½ package (12 ounces) fat-free soy crumbles
  Chili powder
- 1 tablespoon minced onion
- 1 tablespoon olive oil
- ⭐ 1 cup chopped avocado

1. In a 4-quart slow cooker, combine the whole tomatoes, pepper, beans, soy crumbles, chili powder to taste, onion, and oil. Cover and cook on high setting for 4 to 6 hours or on medium setting for 8 hours or until thick. Garnish each serving with ¼ cup avocado.

Makes 4 servings

Per serving: 358 calories, 24 g protein, 34 g carbohydrates, 13.5 g fat, 2 g saturated fat, 0 mg cholesterol, 807 mg sodium, 13 g fiber

Black Bean Chili

Preparation time: 5 minutes | Cooking time: 3 minutes

- 1 cup fat-free soy crumbles
- 1 cup canned, no-salt-added, black beans, rinsed and drained
- 1 cup lower-sodium chipotle-flavored salsa
- 2 teaspoons chili powder
- 1 teaspoon ground cumin
- ½ cup mashed avocado

1. In a saucepan over medium heat, combine the soy crumbles, beans, salsa, chili powder, and cumin. Cook, stirring occasionally, for about 3 minutes, or until heated through. Top each serving with ¼ cup of avocado.

Makes 2 servings

Per serving: 338 calories, 20 g protein, 39 g carbohydrates, 9 fat, 1.7 g saturated fat, 0 mg cholesterol, 674 mg sodium, 15 g fiber

Make It a Flat Belly Diet Meal

Serve with 1 cup sliced red pepper (40)
Total calories: 378

Hearty Country Vegetable Soup

Preparation time: 15 minutes | Cooking time: 2 hours, 15 minutes

- ⭐ ½ **cup olive oil, divided**
- ½ **large onion, chopped**
- 3 **ribs celery, chopped**
- 1 **small head green cabbage, chopped**
- 2 **carrots, chopped**
- 2 **cloves garlic, minced**
- ½ **cup dried white beans**
- 3 **cans (14.5 ounces each) low-sodium vegetable broth**
- 1½ **teaspoons chopped fresh thyme, or ½ teaspoon dried**
- 1½ **teaspoons chopped fresh savory or sage, or ½ teaspoon dried**
- ½ **pound green beans, cut into 1" pieces**
- 1 **zucchini, halved lengthwise and sliced**

1. Heat ¼ cup oil in a soup pot over medium-low heat. Stir in the onion, celery, cabbage, carrots, and garlic. Cover and cook for 12 to 15 minutes, stirring occasionally. Add the beans and 5 cups of the broth. Bring the mixture to a boil. Reduce the heat to medium-low and stir in the thyme and savory. Cover and cook for 1 to 1½ hours, or until the beans are almost tender, adding some of the remaining broth if the soup becomes too thick.

2. Stir in the green beans and zucchini. Partially cover and cook for 20 to 30 minutes, or until the green beans are tender. Divide among 8 bowls. Drizzle ½ tablespoon of the remaining oil in each bowl.

Makes 8 servings

Per serving: 237 calories, 6 g protein, 23 g carbohydrates, 14 g fat, 2 g saturated fat, 0 mg cholesterol, 353 mg sodium, 7 g fiber

Make It a Flat Belly Diet Meal
Serve with 2 cups baby greens (15) and 1 cup halved grape tomatoes (30) tossed with 2 tablespoons Annie's Naturals® Goddess Dressing (90)
Total calories: 372

Turnip and Carrot Soup with Parmesan

Preparation time: 15 minutes | Cooking time: 20 minutes

  1 pound white turnips, peeled and quartered

  4 large carrots, cut into chunks

  2 large red or white new potatoes, quartered

  1 large onion, chopped

  5 cloves garlic, smashed

1½ cups low-sodium chicken broth

1½ cups water

1½ teaspoons chopped fresh thyme, or ½ teaspoon dried

1½ teaspoons chopped fresh sage, or ½ teaspoon dried

¼ teaspoon salt

¼ teaspoon freshly ground black pepper

  1 cup 1% milk

½ cup (2 ounces) grated Parmesan cheese

  1 cup toasted pine nuts

1. In a large saucepan or Dutch oven, combine the turnips, carrots, potatoes, onion, garlic, broth, water, thyme, sage, salt, and pepper. Bring to a boil over high heat. Reduce the heat to medium, cover, and simmer for 20 minutes, or until the vegetables are very tender.

2. In batches, transfer the cooked vegetables into the bowl of a food processor fitted with a metal blade, or into a blender, and puree until smooth. When all the soup has been pureed, return it to the pan. Stir in the milk. Cook over low heat just until heated through (do not boil). Remove from the heat and stir in the Parmesan. Ladle into bowls, top each with 2 tablespoons of pine nuts.

Makes 8 servings

Per serving: 261 calories, 9 g protein, 28 g carbohydrates, 13.5 g fat, 2 g saturated fat, 7 mg cholesterol, 263 mg sodium, 5 g fiber

Make It a Flat Belly Diet Meal

Serve with 2 Laughing Cow® Light Garlic & Herb Cheese wedges (70) and 2 Ry Krisp® crackers (70)

Total calories: 401

Chilled Strawberry Soup

Preparation time: 5 minutes | Cooking time: 4 minutes | Cooling time:
5 minutes | Chilling time: 60 minutes

  2 cups fresh strawberries, hulled
  ¾ cup white grape juice
  ¼ cup orange juice
  ¼ teaspoon lemon extract
  ⅛ teaspoon freshly grated nutmeg
  1 cup fat-free vanilla yogurt
  ½ cup toasted slivered almonds

1. In a 2-quart saucepan, bring the strawberries, grape juice, orange juice, lemon extract, and nutmeg to a boil over medium heat, stirring occasionally. Reduce the heat and simmer for 1 minute. Remove from the heat and allow to cool for 5 minutes.

2. Transfer the soup to a blender and puree until smooth. Pour into a large bowl. Chill for 30 minutes. Whisk in the yogurt and chill another 30 minutes before serving. Divide evenly into 4 bowls, top each with 2 tablespoons almonds.

Makes 4 servings

Per serving: 195 calories, 7 g protein, 28 g carbohydrates, 7 g fat, 0.5 g saturated fat, 1 mg cholesterol, 48 mg sodium, 3 g fiber

Make It a Flat Belly Diet Meal

Serve with 5 Ry Krisp® crackers (175)

Total calories: 370

Cucumber and Melon Salad with Watercress, Herbs, and Feta

Preparation time: 25 minutes

DRESSING

- 2 teaspoons extra virgin olive oil
- 2 tablespoons freshly squeezed lemon juice
- 2 tablespoons white wine vinegar
- 1 tablespoon minced shallot
- 1 teaspoon sugar
- ½ teaspoon salt
- ½ teaspoon freshly ground black pepper

SALAD

- 3 cucumbers, peeled and chopped (about 6 cups)
- 8 cups melon balls (1 honeydew or various types)
- 1 bunch watercress, large stems discarded
- ½ cup fresh mint leaves
- ½ cup crumbled feta cheese
- ½ cup toasted pine nuts
- 1 tablespoon chopped Kalamata olives

1. To prepare the dressing: In a small bowl, whisk together the oil, lemon juice, vinegar, shallot, sugar, salt, and pepper.

2. To prepare the salad: In a large bowl, combine the cucumbers, melon balls, watercress, mint, feta, pine nuts, and olives. Pour the dressing on the salad, toss gently to coat. Divide evenly on 4 plates and serve.

Makes 4 servings

Per serving: 354 calories, 9 g protein, 43 g carbohydrates, 19 g fat, 4 g saturated fat, 17 mg cholesterol, 548 mg sodium, 5 g fiber

Crab Salad with Avocado and Pomelo

Preparation time: 22 minutes

DRESSING

- 2 tablespoons orange juice
- 2 teaspoons extra virgin olive oil
- 2 tablespoons white wine vinegar
- 2 teaspoons finely chopped fresh tarragon or chervil
- ½ teaspoon freshly grated orange zest
- ½ teaspoon salt
- ¼ teaspoon dry mustard
- ¼ teaspoon freshly ground black pepper

SALAD

- 2 heads butterhead lettuce, separated into leaves (about 8 cups)
- 2 medium sweet onions (such as Vidalia), sliced (about 2 cups)
- 2 pomelos, peeled and cut into sections (about 4 cups) (See Note)
- ⭐ 1 cup sliced avocado
- 1 cup lump crabmeat
- 1 tablespoon chopped blanched hazelnuts, toasted

1. To prepare the dressing: In a medium bowl, whisk together the orange juice, oil, vinegar, tarragon or chervil, orange zest, salt, mustard, and pepper.

2. To prepare the salad: In a large bowl, combine the lettuce, onions, and pomelo. Add the dressing and toss to coat. Mound the salad onto 4 plates. Top with avocado slices, ¼ cup of the crabmeat, and hazelnuts.

Makes 4 servings

Per serving: 237 calories, 11 g protein, 31 g carbohydrates, 10 g fat, 1.5 g saturated fat, 30 mg cholesterol, 335 mg sodium, 7 g fiber

Note: Replace the pomelos with grapefruit if they're not available.

Make It a Flat Belly Diet Meal
Serve with 4 Ry Krisp® crackers (140)
Total calories: 377

Curried Barley and Shrimp Salad

Preparation time: 20 minutes | Cooking time: 45 minutes

  3 cups water
  1 teaspoon curry powder
  ½ teaspoon turmeric
  1 cup barley
  ¼ cup plus 1 tablespoon freshly squeezed lime juice (about 4 limes)
  1 tablespoon vegetable oil
  2 teaspoons finely chopped jalapeño chile pepper, seeded (See Note)
  1 clove garlic, minced
  ¼ teaspoon salt
  1 pound small cooked shrimp, peeled and deveined
  1½ cups seeded and diced tomatoes
  ½ cups chopped green bell pepper
  ½ cup chopped peeled cucumber
  12 cups baby greens
  ¼ cup chopped fresh basil
  ¾ cup toasted pumpkin seeds

1. In a large saucepan over high heat, bring the water, curry, and turmeric to a boil. Stir in the barley. Cover and reduce the heat to low. Cook for about 45 minutes, or until the water is absorbed and the barley is tender. Remove from heat. Meanwhile in a large bowl, whisk together the lime juice, oil, chile pepper, garlic, and salt. Add the shrimp, tomatoes, bell pepper, cucumber, and barley. Toss to coat.

2. Spoon the salad on top of 2 cups of baby greens per plate. Divide salad evenly and sprinkle on the basil and pumpkin seeds.

Makes 6 servings

Per serving: 338 calories, 24 g protein, 35 g carbohydrates, 12.5 g fat, 2.5 g saturated fat, 115 mg cholesterol, 273 mg sodium, 7 g fiber

Note: Wear plastic gloves and keep hands away from eyes when handling fresh chile peppers.

Make It a Flat Belly Diet Meal

Serve on a bed of 2 cups baby greens (15)

Total calories: 353

Warm Quinoa Salad

Preparation time: 8 minutes | Cooking time: 10 minutes

- 2 cups water
- 1 cup quinoa, rinsed and drained
- 1 cup chopped radicchio (about ½ head), plus leaves for garnish
- ½ cup chopped fresh cilantro
- ½ cup golden raisins
- ½ cup fat-free honey mustard dressing
- ½ teaspoon salt
  Freshly ground black pepper
- ★ ½ cup toasted chopped cashews

1. In a medium saucepan, over high heat, bring the water and quinoa to a boil. Reduce the heat to a simmer, cover, and cook for about 5 minutes, or until all the liquid is absorbed.

2. Transfer the quinoa to a medium serving bowl. Add the chopped radicchio, cilantro, raisins, dressing, and salt. Toss to coat. Season to taste with pepper. Place the radicchio leaves on 4 plates, divide the salad evenly, and sprinkle each with 2 tablespoons of cashews.

Makes 4 servings

Per serving: 363 calories, 9 g protein, 60 g carbohydrates, 10.5 g fat, 2 g saturated fat, 0 mg cholesterol, 435 mg sodium, 4g fiber

Italian Shrimp and Pasta Salad

Preparation time: 7 minutes | Cooking time: 10 minutes

½ cup whole wheat fusilli pasta
1 can (3 ounces) tiny shrimp, drained
½ cup halved grape tomatoes
¼ cup torn fresh basil
1 teaspoon Italian seasoning
1 teaspoon olive oil
★ ¼ cup toasted pine nuts

1. In a medium pot of rapidly boiling water, cook the pasta for 8 to 10 minutes or until al dente. Drain and rinse with cold water until cool to the touch.

2. In a large bowl, combine the shrimp, tomatoes, basil, Italian seasoning, oil, and pasta. Toss to coat and sprinkle with the nuts.

Makes 2 servings

Per serving: 231 calories, 12 g protein, 15 g carbohydrates, 15 g fat, 1 g saturated fat, 87 mg cholesterol, 362 mg sodium, 3 g fiber

Make It a Flat Belly Diet Meal
Serve with 1 string cheese (80) and 1 cups grapes (60)
Total calories: 371

Turkey-Avocado Cobb Salad

Preparation time: 8 minutes | Cooking time: 7 minutes

1 pound turkey breast cutlets

2 teaspoons olive oil, plus 1 teaspoon for the turkey

2 tablespoons cider vinegar

1 tablespoon water

1 teaspoon Dijon mustard

8 cups baby spinach

4 slices cooked turkey bacon, chopped

1 cup diced avocado

4 cherry tomatoes, halved

1 ounce blue cheese, crumbled

   Freshly ground black pepper

1. Preheat a grill pan on medium-high heat for 2 minutes. Brush the turkey with 1 teaspoon of the oil. Grill the turkey for 4 minutes, flip, and continue cooking for about 3 minutes longer, or until centers are opaque. Cut into chunks.

2. In a glass jar, combine the vinegar, water, mustard, and the remaining 2 teaspoons oil. Cover and shake well.

3. In a large bowl, combine the spinach with 2 tablespoons of the dressing. Toss to coat the leaves. Arrange the turkey, bacon, avocados, tomatoes, and cheese over the spinach. Drizzle on the remaining dressing, and season with black pepper to taste.

Makes 4 servings

Per serving: 288 calories, 34 g protein, 10 g carbohydrates, 13.5 g fat, 3.1 g saturated fat, 57 mg cholesterol, 473 mg sodium, 5 g fiber

Make It a Flat Belly Diet Meal

Serve with 1 medium apple (80)

Total calories: 368

Soba Noodle Salad with Snow Peas

Preparation time: 15 minutes

- 8 ounces dry soba noodles or whole wheat spaghetti
- 2 tablespoons honey
- 2 tablespoons freshly squeezed lime juice (about 2 limes)
- 2 tablespoons rice wine vinegar
- 2 tablespoons reduced-sodium soy sauce
- 1 tablespoon grated fresh ginger
- ¼ teaspoon red pepper flakes
- 2 tablespoons peanut oil
- 2 cups shredded cooked chicken
- 2 cups julienned fresh snow peas
- 2 red bell peppers, seeded and thinly sliced lengthwise
- 1 cup grated carrots
- 1½ cups diced avocado
- ¼ cup fresh cilantro, coarsely chopped

1. Cook the noodles according to the package directions. Drain and rinse with cold water. Set aside.

2. In a large bowl, whisk together the honey, lime juice, vinegar, soy sauce, ginger, and pepper flakes. Whisk in the oil in a steady stream.

3. Fold in the chicken, snow peas, bell peppers, carrots, avocado, cilantro, and noodles.

Makes 6 servings

Per serving: 352 calories, 20 g protein, 48 g carbohydrates, 11 g fat, 2 g saturated fat, 26 mg cholesterol, 392 mg sodium, 6 g fiber

Spinach Salad

Preparation time: 8 minutes

  2 tablespoons balsamic vinegar

  1 tablespoon olive oil

 ⅛ teaspoon freshly ground black pepper

  3 cups fresh baby spinach leaves

 ¼ cup sliced mushrooms

 ¼ cup halved yellow grape tomatoes

  1 small red bell pepper, seeded and sliced into strips

1. In a salad or pasta bowl, whisk together the vinegar, oil, and black pepper. Add the spinach and toss to coat. Top with the mushrooms, tomatoes, and bell pepper.

Makes 1 serving

Per serving: 209 calories, 4 g protein, 20 g carbohydrates, 14 g fat, 2 g saturated fat, 0 mg cholesterol, 353 mg sodium, 6 g fiber

Make It a Flat Belly Diet Meal

Serve with 4 Ry Krisp® crackers (105) and 2 Laughing Cow® Light Garlic & Herb wedges (70)

Total calories: 384

Herb and Mesclun Salad with Grilled Shrimp

Preparation time: 30 minutes | Marinating time: 20 minutes | Cooking time: 4 minutes

¼ cup fresh lime juice, divided (about 4 limes)
½ teaspoon ground cumin, divided
¼ teaspoon salt, divided
¼ teaspoon red pepper flakes, divided
1 pound large shrimp, peeled and deveined
6 cups mixed baby greens
1 cup fresh mint
1 cup fresh cilantro
1 cup fresh flat-leaf parsley
1 small red onion, thinly sliced
2 tablespoons vegetable oil
½ cup toasted slivered almonds

1. In medium bowl, whisk together 2 tablespoons of the lime juice, ¼ teaspoon of the cumin, ⅛ teaspoon of the salt, and a pinch of the pepper flakes. Stir in the shrimp and chill for 20 minutes.

2. Meanwhile, in a serving bowl, toss together the baby greens, mint, cilantro, parsley, and onion. Chill until ready to serve.

3. In a small bowl, whisk together the oil, ¼ teaspoon cumin, ⅛ teaspoon salt, the remaining pepper flakes, and 2 tablespoons of the lime juice.

4. Grill or broil the shrimp for about 2 minutes each side, or until just opaque. Add the shrimp and dressing to the greens. Toss gently to coat. Divide evenly on 4 plates and top with the almonds.

Makes 4 servings

Per serving: 280 calories, 25 g protein, 11 g carbohydrates, 16 g fat, 1.5 g saturated fat, 151 mg cholesterol, 327 mg sodium, 5 g fiber

Make It a Flat Belly Diet Meal

Serve with ½ Thomas'® Multigrain Sahara Pita (70) and 2 tablespoons hummus (50)

Total calories: 400

Curried Potato Salad

Preparation time: 10 minutes

- 1 pound potatoes, boiled and cubed
- 2 scallions, chopped
- ½ cup toasted sliced almonds
- ¼ cup raisins
- ½ cup fat-free plain yogurt
- 2 tablespoons mango chutney
- 2 teaspoons curry powder

1. Place the potatoes in a large bowl and stir in the scallions, almonds, and raisins.

2. In a small bowl, whisk together the yogurt, chutney, and curry powder. Pour over the potatoes and toss to combine well. Divide evenly onto 4 plates and serve.

Makes 4 servings

Per serving: 226 calories, 6 g protein, 39 g carbohydrates, 6.5 g fat, 0.5 g saturated fat, 1 mg cholesterol, 26 mg sodium, 4 g dietary fiber

Make It a Flat Belly Diet Meal

Serve on a bed of 2 cups baby greens (15) with 3 ounces grilled chicken breast (90) and 1 medium apple (80)

Total calories: 411

Bitter Greens with Hot Vinaigrette Dressing

Preparation time: 5 minutes | Cooking time: 7 minutes

½ cup balsamic vinegar

2 teaspoons honey

1 teaspoon Dijon mustard

2 cloves garlic, minced

1½ teaspoons chopped fresh tarragon, or ½ teaspoon dried

⅛ teaspoon freshly ground black pepper

4 cups torn bitter greens, such as dandelion

2 slices turkey bacon, cooked until crisp and crumbled

★ ½ cup toasted pine nuts

1. Arrange the greens on 4 salad plates.

2. In a 1-quart saucepan, whisk together the vinegar, honey, mustard, garlic, tarragon, and pepper. Cook over medium heat for 1 to 2 minutes, or until the mixture is hot but not boiling.

3. Spoon immediately over the greens and toss well to coat. Sprinkle each salad evenly with bacon and pine nuts.

Makes 4 servings

Per serving: 198 calories, 5 g protein, 18 g carbohydrates, 13 g fat, 2 g saturated fat, 8 mg cholesterol, 141 mg sodium, 2 g fiber

Make It a Flat Belly Diet Meal

Serve with 3 ounces grilled pork tenderloin (115) and ¼ cup steamed brown rice (55)

Total calories: 368

Moroccan Carrot Salad with Toasted Cumin

Preparation time: 10 minutes | Cooking time: 2 minutes

- ¾ teaspoon ground cumin
- ¼ teaspoon ground coriander
- ½ cup reduced-fat sour cream
- ¼ cup flaxseed oil
- 1 tablespoon plus 1 teaspoon lemon juice (about 1 lemon)
- 1½ teaspoons extra virgin olive oil
- ¼ teaspoon freshly grated orange zest
- ¼ teaspoon salt
- 7 medium carrots, peeled and grated
- ½ cup currants
- 2 tablespoons finely chopped red onion

1. In a small dry skillet over medium heat, toast the cumin and coriander, stirring often, for 2 minutes or until fragrant and slightly darker in color. Place in a medium bowl and let cool. Stir in the sour cream, flaxseed oil, lemon juice, olive oil, orange zest, and salt.

2. Add the carrots, currants, and onion, and toss to coat well. Divide evenly on 4 plates.

Makes 4 servings

Per serving: 276 calories, 3 g protein, 26 g carbohydrates, 19.5 g fat, 4 g saturated fat, 12 mg cholesterol, 234 mg sodium, 4 g fiber

Make It a Flat Belly Diet Meal

Serve with 3 ounces broiled medium shrimp (90)

Total calories: 366

Spinach Salad with Radishes and Walnuts

Preparation time: 10 minutes

- 1 tablespoon freshly squeezed lemon juice (about 1 lemon)
- 2 teaspoons white wine vinegar
- Salt
- Freshly ground black pepper
- ¼ cup extra virgin olive oil
- 5 ounces baby spinach leaves
- 4 medium radishes, thinly sliced
- ½ cup walnut halves

1. In a large bowl, whisk together the lemon juice and vinegar. Season to taste with salt and pepper. Whisk in the olive oil slowly.

2. When ready to serve, toss together the spinach and radishes and toss with the dressing to coat. Divide evenly on 4 salad plates, sprinkle each with 2 tablespoons of the walnuts.

Makes 4 servings

Per serving: 224 calories, 3 g protein, 6 g carbohydrates, 22 g fat, 2.5 g saturated fat, 0 mg cholesterol, 204 mg sodium, 3 g fiber

Make It a Flat Belly Diet Meal

Serve with 3 ounces chunk light tuna in water, drained (120) and 1½ cups grapes (60)

Total calories: 404

Strawberry and Red Onion Salad

Preparation time: 10 minutes | Standing time: 15 minutes

  3 tablespoons strawberry all-fruit spread
  2 teaspoons balsamic vinegar
  1 teaspoon olive oil
  1 teaspoon flaxseed oil
  ⅛ teaspoon salt
  ⅛ teaspoon red pepper flakes
  1 pound fresh strawberries, hulled and halved
  ¼ cantaloupe, cut into cubes
  ½ small red bell pepper, seeded and diced
  ½ small red onion, thinly sliced
  1 medium head escarole, torn in pieces
  1 cup diced avocado
    Freshly ground black pepper

1. In a medium bowl, combine the all-fruit spread, vinegar, olive oil, flaxseed oil, salt, and red pepper flakes until well blended. Gently fold in the strawberries, cantaloupe, bell pepper, and onion. Cover and let stand for 15 minutes to allow the flavors to blend.

2. Place the escarole in a serving bowl. Add the avocado and the strawberry mixture and toss to coat. Season with black pepper to taste, and divide evenly on 4 plates.

Makes 4 servings

Per serving: 186 calories, 4 g protein, 28 g carbohydrates, 8.5 g fat, 1 g saturated fat, 0 mg cholesterol, 111 mg sodium, 9 g fiber

Make It a Flat Belly Diet Meal

Serve with 3 ounces grilled chicken breast (90) and ⅔ cup frozen Cascadian Farm® Edamame, thawed (120)

Total calories: 396

Crisp Romaine Salad with Chicken and Mango

Preparation time: 25 minutes | Cooking time: 15 minutes

  2 tablespoons olive oil, divided
  3 boneless, skinless chicken breast halves, trimmed (6 ounces each)
 ½ teaspoon salt, divided
 ¼ teaspoon freshly ground black pepper, divided
  2 shallots, finely chopped
  2 tablespoons balsamic vinegar, divided
  4 cups shredded romaine lettuce
  1 small bunch watercress, large stems discarded
 ½ cup finely shredded red cabbage
  1 firm ripe mango, pitted, peeled, and cut into ½" pieces
 ½ cup toasted pumpkin seeds

1. Heat 1 tablespoon oil in a large nonstick skillet over medium heat. Season both sides of the chicken with ¼ teaspoon salt and ⅛ teaspoon pepper. Cook, turning once, until cooked through, about 6 minutes on each side. Transfer to a plate; cover and chill completely.

2. Add the shallots and 1 tablespoon vinegar to the skillet and cook, stirring, for about 3 minutes, or until the liquid is almost evaporated. Transfer to a small bowl. Whisk in the remaining 1 tablespoon oil, 1 tablespoon vinegar, ¼ teaspoon salt, and ⅛ teaspoon pepper.

3. In a serving bowl, toss together the romaine, watercress, cabbage, and mango. Cut the chicken diagonally into long, thin strips. Add to the romaine mixture, and toss with dressing and pumpkin seeds.

Makes 4 servings

Per serving: 301 calories, 33 g protein, 19 g carbohydrates, 10.5 g fat, 2 g saturated fat, 74 mg cholesterol, 384 mg sodium, 3 g fiber

Make It a Flat Belly Diet Meal
Serve with 3 Ry Krisp® crackers (105)
Total calories: 406

Greek Lemon Chicken

Preparation time: 18 minutes | Cooking time: 45 minutes

4	skinless, split, bone-in chicken breasts, trimmed (about 1½ pounds)
1	medium red bell pepper, seeded and cut into 8 wedges
1	medium orange bell pepper, seeded and cut into 8 wedges
1	medium Yukon gold potato, cut into 8 wedges
1	medium red onion, peeled and cut into 8 wedges
★ 40	pitted Kalamata olives, smashed (about 1⅓ cups)
1	tablespoon extra virgin olive oil
	Grated zest and juice of 1 lemon
1	tablespoon minced garlic
1	tablespoon chopped fresh oregano, or 1 teaspoon dried
¾	teaspoon freshly ground black pepper
¾	teaspoon paprika

1. Preheat the oven to 400°F.

2. Tear off 2 sheets of nonstick aluminum foil, each 24" long. Put dull sides (nonstick sides) together, and fold over the edge on one side twice, to make a seam. Open up, and line and cover the edges of a 17" by 12" rimmed baking pan (the dull side of the foil should face up).

3. Place the chicken on one side of the pan and the bell peppers, potatoes, onion, and olives on the other. In a bowl, whisk together the oil, lemon zest and juice, garlic, oregano, salt, black pepper, and paprika. Drizzle over the chicken and vegetables, and toss to coat.

4. Roast for 40 to 45 minutes, turning the chicken and stirring the vegetables halfway through cooking, or until a meat thermometer registers 165°F when inserted into the thickest part of the chicken (not touching bone). Arrange 1 chicken breast and ¼ of the vegetables on 4 plates.

Makes 4 servings

Per serving: 401 calories, 39 g protein, 19 g carbohydrates, 18 g fat, 2.5 g saturated fat, 115 mg cholesterol, 742 mg sodium, 3 g fiber

Spinach-Stuffed Chicken Roulade

Preparation time: 8 minutes | Cooking time: 25 minutes

- ¼ cup finely chopped onion
- 1 clove garlic, minced
- ¼ teaspoon red pepper flakes (or to taste)
- 2 teaspoons olive oil, divided
- 1 tablespoon water
- ¼ cup grated Parmesan cheese
- 1 package (10 ounces) frozen chopped spinach, thawed, drained, and squeezed dry
- 4 chicken breast cutlets (about 1 pound)
- 2 tablespoons minced dry-packed sun-dried tomatoes
- ½ cup low-sodium chicken broth
- ½ cup toasted pine nuts

1. In a medium nonstick skillet over medium heat, cook the onion, garlic, and pepper flakes in 1 teaspoon oil for 30 seconds. Reduce the heat to low, cover, and cook, stirring once, for about 3 minutes, until softened. In a small bowl, combine the onion mixture, Parmesan, and spinach.

2. Lay the chicken on a work surface, smooth side down. Sprinkle the tomatoes evenly on the chicken. Divide the spinach mixture evenly among the cutlets. Pat the mixture to edges of 3 sides, leaving about 1" at the narrow tip free of spinach. Loosely roll up the cutlet, ending with narrow tip, and secure with wooden picks.

3. Add the remaining 1 teaspoon oil to the skillet set over medium heat. Add the chicken and cook about 10 minutes or until golden brown on all sides. Add the broth. Cover and cook over low heat for about 7 minutes or until cooked through. Transfer the roulades to a serving platter. Cover with aluminum foil to keep warm. Boil the juices in skillet for about 5 minutes. Cut the roulades into diagonal slices. Drizzle with the pan juices and sprinkle with the nuts.

Makes 4 servings

Per serving: 322 calories, 33 g protein, 8 g carbohydrates, 17 g fat, 2.5 g saturated fat, 70 mg cholesterol, 302 mg sodium, 2 g fiber

Make It a Flat Belly Diet Meal

Serve with 1 medium orange (70)
Total calories: 392

Chicken with Citrus-Avocado Salsa

Preparation time: 8 minutes | Cooking time: 15 minutes

4　boneless, skinless chicken breast halves (about 1½ pounds)

4　cups water

½　teaspoon plus ⅛ teaspoon salt

1　ruby red grapefruit

1　cup diced avocado

4　radishes, thinly sliced

¼　cup chopped basil leaves

Fresh basil (optional)

1. In a large saucepan, combine the chicken, water, and ½ teaspoon salt. Cover and bring to a boil over high heat. Turn off the heat and let sit for 15 minutes, or until a thermometer inserted in the thickest portion registers 165°F.

2. Meanwhile, with a knife, remove the peel and pith from the grapefruit. Working over a bowl to catch the juice, free each segment from its membrane and cut the segments into bite-size pieces, dropping them into the bowl. Add the avocado, radishes, basil, and the remaining ⅛ teaspoon salt. Gently toss to mix.

3. Drain the chicken breasts, discarding the liquid. Cut crosswise into ½" slices. Divide the grapefruit mixture onto 4 plates and add a ¼ of the chicken to each, drizzling the chicken with juice from mixture. Garnish with basil leaves, if using.

Makes 4 servings

Per serving: 269 calories, 41 g protein, 9 g carbohydrates, 7.5 g fat, 1.5 g saturated fat, 99 mg cholesterol, 188 mg sodium, 3 g fiber

Make It a Flat Belly Diet Meal

Serve with ½ cup steamed brown rice (108)

Total calories: 377

Grilled Ginger-Soy Chicken

Preparation time: 10 minutes | Marinating time: 2 hours | Cooking time: 20 minutes

¼ cup reduced-sodium soy sauce

2 tablespoons minced fresh ginger

2 tablespoons honey

2 tablespoons miso paste

1 tablespoon minced garlic

2 teaspoons toasted sesame oil

¼ teaspoon red pepper flakes

8 boneless, skinless chicken breast halves (3-4 pounds total)

½ teaspoon kosher salt

⭐ 1 cup unsalted dry-roasted peanuts halves

1. In a large resealable plastic storage bag, combine the first seven ingredients. Add the chicken, and turn to coat. Seal and chill for at least 2 hours.

2. Lightly coat a grill rack with vegetable oil spray. Heat the grill to medium for indirect heat. (If using a charcoal grill, position the coals on one half of grill. If using a gas grill, heat one side to high, the other to low.)

3. Remove the chicken from the marinade. Discard the marinade. Season the chicken with kosher salt.

4. Place the chicken on the hottest section of the grill. Cook for 10 minutes turning once. Move to the cooler section of the grill and cook 10 minutes, or until a thermometer inserted into the thickest part of the chicken registers 165°F. Sprinkle with peanuts.

Makes 8 servings

Per serving: 317 calories, 44 g protein, 8 g carbohydrates, 12 g fat, 2 g saturated fat, 99 mg cholesterol, 424 mg sodium, 2 g fiber

Make It a Flat Belly Diet Meal

Serve with 1 cup sliced red peppers (40) with 2 tablespoons hummus for dipping (50)

Total calories: 407

Grilled Oregano Chicken

Preparation time: 10 minutes | Marinating time: 2 hours | Cooking time: 17 minutes

    6 small boneless, skinless chicken breast halves (about 2¼ pounds)
    1 cup coarsely chopped fresh oregano leaves
    4 scallions, trimmed and thinly sliced
    ½ cup balsamic vinegar
    ⅓ cup extra virgin olive oil
    2 teaspoons freshly ground black pepper
    ¾ teaspoon salt

1. Place the chicken breast halves between 2 sheets of plastic wrap. Using a mallet or heavy pan, pound to ¾" thickness.

2. In a plastic resealable food storage bag, combine the oregano, scallions, vinegar, oil, pepper, and salt. Add the chicken, seal, and turn to coat. Chill for 2 hours.

3. Lightly coat a grill rack with nonstick cooking spray. Preheat the grill to medium for indirect heat. (If using a charcoal grill, position the coals on one half of the grill. If using a gas grill, heat one side to high, the other to low.)

4. Remove the chicken from the marinade, reserving the marinade. Place the chicken on the hottest section of the grill. Cook for 6 minutes, turning once. Move the chicken to the cooler section of the grill and cook for 6 minutes more, turning once, until a thermometer inserted into the thickest part of the breast registers 165°F.

Makes 6 servings

Per serving: 317 calories, 40 g protein, 5 g carbohydrates, 15 g fat, 2 g saturated fat, 99 mg cholesterol, 410 mg sodium, 0 g fiber

Make It a Flat Belly Diet Meal

Serve with 1 cup grape tomatoes (30) and 1 Laughing Cow® Light Garlic & Herb wedge (35)

Total calories: 382

Lime-Marinated Chicken with Salsa

Preparation time: 20 minutes | Marinating time: 1 hour |
Cooking time: 13 to 15 minutes

- 4 boneless, skinless chicken breast halves (about 1¼ pounds)
- 3 tablespoons lime juice (about 3 limes)
- 2 tablespoons olive oil
- 1¼ teaspoons ground cumin
- ¼ teaspoon kosher salt
- 3 medium tomatoes, chopped
- 1 cup chopped avocado
- ½ cup chopped sweet onion (such as Vidalia)
- ½ cup chopped fresh cilantr
- 1 small jalapeño chile pepper, seeded and finely chopped (see Note)

1. Put the chicken into a large resealable plastic bag.

2. In a small bowl, whisk the lime juice, oil, cumin, and salt. Transfer 2 tablespoons of the marinade to a medium glass bowl and cover with plastic wrap. Pour the remaining marinade into the chicken bag. Seal and turn to coat. Chill for at least 1 hour.

3. Meanwhile add the tomatoes, avocado, onion, chopped cilantro, and chile pepper to the bowl with the lime marinade. Toss gently to mix. Cover the salsa and chill.

4. Coat the grill rack or broiler pan with nonstick cooking spray. Preheat the grill to medium-high for direct heat, or the broiler to 450°F. Cook the chicken for 6 minutes on each side or until a thermometer inserted into thickest part of the chicken registers 165°F.

Makes 4 servings

Per serving: 307 calories, 35 g protein, 10 g carbohydrates, 14.5 g fat, 2 g saturated fat, 82 mg cholesterol, 249 mg sodium, 4 g fiber

Note: Wear plastic gloves and keep hands away from eyes when handling fresh chile peppers.

Make It a Flat Belly Diet Meal

Serve on a bed of 2 cups baby greens (15) and 2 Ry Krisp® crackers (70)
Total calories: 392

Grape-ful Chicken

Preparation time: 15 minutes | Cooking time: 35 minutes

- 1 small butternut squash, peeled, seeded, and cut into 1" cubes
- 1 cup pearl onions, peeled
- 4 skinless, bone-in chicken breast halves (about 1 pound)
- ¼ teaspoon salt
- ¼ teaspoon freshly ground black pepper
- ¼ cup chopped fresh tarragon
- 2 teaspoons olive oil
- 1½ cups low-sodium chicken broth, divided
- 1 tablespoon cornstarch
- 2 cups seedless red grapes
- ⭐ ½ cup toasted chopped walnuts

1. Place the squash cubes on a microwaveable plate and sprinkle them with water to moisten. Microwave on high power for 4 minutes.

2. Season both sides of the chicken with the salt and pepper, and rub with the tarragon.

3. Heat the oil in a large Dutch oven over medium-high heat. Add the chicken, and cook for 3 minutes per side, or until golden brown. Add the squash, onions, and 1 cup of the broth, and bring to a simmer. Reduce the heat to medium, cover, and cook for 15 minutes.

4. Using a slotted spoon, transfer the chicken and vegetables to a serving platter, reserving the liquid in the pot.

5. Dissolve the cornstarch in the remaining ½ cup chicken broth. Whisk the mixture into the remaining liquid in the pot. Simmer, whisking, for 1 to 2 minutes, or until the liquid thickens. Add the grapes. Simmer for 1 minute. Spoon the sauce over the chicken and vegetables. Sprinkle with the walnuts, and serve immediately.

Makes 4 servings

Per serving: 397 calories, 34 g protein, 38 g carbohydrates, 14 g fat, 2 g saturated fat, 68 mg cholesterol, 264 mg sodium, 4 g fiber

Almond-Encrusted Chicken Breast

Preparation time: 5 minutes | Cooking time: 10 minutes

  5 ounces boneless, skinless chicken breast
  1 tablespoon cornstarch
  ¼ cup fat-free egg substitute
  2 tablespoons finely chopped almonds

1. Sprinkle each side of the chicken breast with cornstarch. Dip the breast into the egg substitute to coat and then sprinkle with almonds.

2. Coat a small nonstick skillet with nonstick cooking spray and heat over medium heat. Cook the chicken 5 minutes on each side or until a thermometer inserted in the thickest part registers 165°F.

Makes 1 serving

Per serving: 310 calories, 43 g protein, 10 g carbohydrates, 9.8 g fat, 1.5 g saturated fat, 83 mg cholesterol, 204 mg sodium, 1 g fiber

Make It a Flat Belly Diet Meal

Serve with ¼ cup nonfat cottage cheese (40) and 1 cup grape tomatoes (30)
Total calories: 380

Chicken with Orange Almond Topping

Preparation time: 10 minutes

- 7 ounces boneless, skinless cooked chicken breasts or cooked chicken pieces, or canned chicken
- ½ cup mandarin orange segments in light syrup, drained
- 2 tablespoons orange marmalade
- 1 tablespoon low-fat red wine vinaigrette
- Pinch of ground allspice
- ¼ cup toasted slivered almonds
- 1 tablespoon chopped scallions

1. Cut the chicken breasts into thin diagonal slices. Fan the slices out on 2 salad plates. If using precooked chicken, cut into bite-size pieces. If using canned chicken, crumble into bite-size pieces.

2. In a small bowl, combine the orange segments, marmalade, vinaigrette, and all-spice. Stir to mix well and spoon over the chicken. Sprinkle on the almonds and scallions.

Makes 2 servings

Per serving: 342 calories, 34 g protein, 27 g carbohydrates, 11.5 g fat, 1.5 g saturated fat, 84 mg cholesterol, 169 mg sodium, 2 g fiber

Make It a Flat Belly Diet Meal

Serve on a bed of 2 cups baby greens (15)

Total calories: 357

Chicken with Banana Chutney Topping

Preparation time: 10 minutes

7   ounces boneless, skinless cooked chicken breasts or cooked chicken pieces,
    or canned chicken
½   medium banana, chopped
2   tablespoons mango chutney
¼   cup toasted chopped cashews
½   teaspoon freshly squeezed lemon juice (about ½ lemon)

1. Cut the chicken breasts into thin diagonal slices. Fan the slices out on 2 salad plates. If using precooked chicken, cut into bite-size pieces. If using canned chicken, crumble into bite-size pieces.

2. In a small bowl, combine the banana, chutney, cashews, and lemon juice. Stir gently to mix. Spoon over the chicken.

Makes 2 servings

Per serving: 337 calories, 34 g protein, 24 g carbohydrates, 11.5 g fat, 2.5 g saturated fat, 84 mg cholesterol, 406 mg sodium, 1 g fiber

Make It a Flat Belly Diet Meal

Serve on a bed of 2 cups baby greens (15)

Total calories: 354

Chicken with Raspberry Topping

Preparation time: 10 minutes

- 7 ounces boneless, skinless cooked chicken breasts or cooked chicken pieces, or canned chicken
- 1 cup fresh raspberries
- 2 tablespoons low-fat raspberry vinaigrette
- ½ teaspoon freshly squeezed lemon juice (about ½ lemon)
- ¼ cup toasted chopped walnuts

1. Cut the chicken breasts into thin diagonal slices. Fan the slices out on 2 salad plates. If using precooked chicken, cut into bite-size pieces. If using canned chicken, crumble into bite-size pieces.

2. In a small bowl, combine the raspberries, vinaigrette, and lemon juice. Spoon over the chicken. Sprinkle with the walnuts.

Makes 2 servings

Per serving: 305 calories, 34 g protein, 13 g carbohydrates, 14.5 g fat, 2 g saturated fat, 84 mg cholesterol, 154 mg sodium, 5 g fiber

Make It a Flat Belly Diet Meal
Serve with ¼ cup steamed wild rice (75)
Total calories: 380

Chicken with Honey Mustard and Pecan Topping

Preparation time: 10 minutes

- 7 ounces boneless, skinless cooked chicken breasts or cooked chicken pieces, or canned chicken
- 2 tablespoons reduced-fat sour cream
- 4 teaspoons honey mustard
- ¼ cup toasted chopped pecans

1. Cut the chicken breasts into thin diagonal slices. Fan the slices out on 2 salad plates. If using precooked chicken, cut into bite-size pieces. If using canned chicken, crumble into bite-size pieces.

2. In a small bowl, combine the sour cream and mustard. Stir to mix well. Dollop onto the chicken. Sprinkle with the pecans.

Makes 2 servings

Per serving: 307 calories, 33 g protein, 5 g carbohydrates, 16 g fat, 3 g saturated fat, 90 mg cholesterol, 120 mg sodium, 1 g fiber

Make It a Flat Belly Diet Meal

Serve on a bed of baby greens (15) with 2 Ry Krisp® crackers (70)
Total calories: 392

Zesty Chicken Fiesta

Preparation time: 5 minutes | Cooking time: 10 minutes

2 cups cooked chicken breast chunks (about 10 to 12 ounces)

1 can (15 ounces) low-sodium black beans, rinsed and drained

1 can (14 ounces) no-salt-added diced tomatoes (with juice)

1 tablespoon chili powder

★ 1 cup chopped avocado

¼ cup fat-free sour cream

1. In a nonstick skillet, combine the chicken, beans, tomatoes, and chili powder. Bring the mixture to a simmer over medium high heat. Reduce the heat to medium and cook, stirring occasionally, for about 5 minutes. Divide onto 4 salad plates, top each with ¼ cup avocado and 1 tablespoon of sour cream.

Makes 4 servings

Per serving: 298 calories, 30 g protein, 26 g carbohydrates, 8.5 g fat, 1.5 g saturated fat, 61 mg cholesterol, 137 mg sodium, 10 g fiber

Make It a Flat Belly Diet Meal

Serve with 1 cup sliced red bell pepper (40) and 2 tablespoons hummus (50)
Total calories: 388

Tuscan Chicken with Beans

Preparation time: 5 minutes

- 1 cup cooked, chopped chicken breast (about 6 ounces)
- 1 cup low-sodium diced tomatoes flavored with garlic and onion, drained
- ⅔ cup no-salt-added canned white beans, rinsed and drained
- 2 teaspoons balsamic vinegar
- 1 cup salad greens
- ¼ cup toasted slivered almonds

1. In a bowl, toss together the chicken, tomatoes, beans, and vinegar.

2. Divide the greens onto 2 salad plates and top each with ½ of the chicken mixture. Serve over greens. Sprinkle with the almonds.

Makes 2 servings

Per serving: 294 calories, 29 g protein, 25 g carbohydrates, 9.5 g fat, 1 g saturated fat, 54 mg cholesterol, 112 mg sodium, 9 g fiber

Make It a Flat Belly Diet Meal

Serve with ¼ cup steamed wild rice (75)
Total calories: 369

Hearty Brussels Sprouts with Sausage

Preparation time: 9 minutes | Cooking time: 24 minutes

  1 **pound low-fat Italian turkey sausage (garlic or mild)**

  2 **teaspoons olive oil**

  ½ **cup toasted slivered almonds**

  6 **whole cardamom pods, cracked**

  ¼ **teaspoon ground cloves**

  ¼ **teaspoon whole cumin seed**

  ⅛ **teaspoon ground white pepper**

1½ **pounds Brussels sprouts, trimmed and quartered**

  ½ **cup low-sodium chicken broth**

1. Remove the sausage from the casings and discard the casings. Crumble the sausage meat with a fork.

2. Warm the oil in 12" skillet over high heat. Add the sausage, almonds, cardamom, cloves, cumin, and pepper. Cook, stirring, for about 6 minutes, or until the sausage and almonds become golden in places.

3. Add the Brussels sprouts and broth. Stir to combine. Cover tightly and cook for 15 minutes, or until the sprouts are tender. Uncover and continue cooking for about 3 minutes, or until most of the liquid in the pan has evaporated. Divide evenly on 4 plates.

Makes 4 servings

Per serving: 341 calories, 33 g protein, 19 g carbohydrates, 17 g fat, 2.9 g saturated fat, 35 mg cholesterol, 54 mg sodium, 8 g fiber

Make It a Flat Belly Diet Meal

Serve on a bed of 2 cups baby greens (15)

Total calories: 356

Steamed Salmon with Snow Peas
Preparation time: 10 minutes | Cooking time: 12 minutes

- 4 skinless salmon fillets, about 1½" thick (about 1 to 1½ pounds)
- 1 teaspoon grated fresh ginger
- 1 clove garlic, minced
- 1 tablespoon freshly squeezed lime juice (about 2 limes)
- 2 teaspoons reduced-sodium soy sauce
- 1 teaspoon toasted sesame oil
- 2 scallions, thinly sliced
- 1 pound snow peas, trimmed
- ★ 1 cup chopped avocado

1. Rub the fillets with the ginger and garlic. Coat a steamer basket with nonstick cooking spray and arrange the fillets in the basket.

2. In a saucepan, bring 2" of water to a boil. Place the steamer basket in the saucepan and cover. Cook for 8 minutes.

3. Meanwhile, in a small bowl, whisk together the lime juice, soy sauce, oil, and scallions. Set aside.

4. After the salmon has cooked for 8 minutes, top with the snow peas and cover. Cook for about 4 minutes, until the salmon is opaque and the snow peas are crisp-tender.

5. Make a bed of the snow peas on 4 plates, top with the salmon, sprinkle with the avocado, drizzle with the reserved sauce.

Makes 4 servings

Per serving: 330 calories, 27 g protein, 13 g carbohydrates, 19 g fat, 3.5 g saturated fat, 67 mg cholesterol, 176 mg sodium, 6 g fiber

Make It a Flat Belly Diet Meal
Serve with 1 medium orange (70)
Total calories: 400

Fish with Summer Squash

Preparation time: 8 minutes | Cooking time: 40 minutes

- 1 large red onion, chopped, divided
- ¼ cup extra virgin olive oil, divided
- 1 strip lemon zest, cut into thin slivers
- 8 ounces zucchini, cut into ½" chunks
- 8 ounces yellow squash, cut into ½" chunks
- 1 clove garlic, minced
- 4 striped bass fillets, about 1" thick (about 1 to 1½ pounds)
- 1 tablespoon red wine vinegar
- 1 tablespoon water
- 2 tablespoons finely chopped fresh mint

1. Preheat the oven to 400°F. Place 2 tablespoons of the onion in a small bowl; set aside. Place the remaining onion in a 13" by 9" baking dish. Add 2 tablespoons of the oil and the lemon zest. Toss and then spread in even layer. Roast, stirring occasionally, for about 15 minutes or until the onion is tender. Remove the baking dish from the oven. Stir in the zucchini, squash, and garlic. Return the dish to the oven and roast for 10 minutes. Remove from the oven.

2. Increase the oven temperature to 450°F. Push the vegetables to one side of the baking dish and add the fish. Arrange the fish evenly in the pan. Spoon the vegetables over the fish. Roast until the fish flakes easily with a fork (8 to 10 minutes for thin fillets and 12 to 15 minutes for thicker fillets).

3. Meanwhile, add the vinegar, water, mint, and the remaining 2 tablespoons oil to the reserved 2 tablespoons of the onion. Place the fillets on 4 plates, spoon the sauce over the fish.

Makes 4 servings

Per serving: 272 calories, 22 g protein, 8 g carbohydrates, 17 g fat, 2.5 g saturated fat, 91 mg cholesterol, 125 mg sodium, 2 g fiber

Make It a Flat Belly Diet Meal

Serve with ¼ cup steamed wild rice (75)
Total calories: 347

Roasted Fish with Artichokes

Preparation time: 10 minutes | Cooking time: 40 to 50 minutes

- 2 large red onions, cut into ¼" wedges
- ¼ cup extra virgin olive oil
- 1 package (10 ounces) frozen artichoke hearts, thawed (about 2 cups)
- 1 cup small cherry or grape tomatoes
- 2 tablespoons chopped parsley
- 1 teaspoon freshly grated orange zest
- 1 clove garlic, minced
- 4 skinless flounder fillets (1–1½ pounds total)

1. Preheat the oven to 400°F.

2. In a 13" by 9" baking dish, combine the onions and oil. Toss and then spread in an even layer.

3. Roast for about 35 minutes, or until the onions are golden. Remove from the oven and stir in the artichokes and tomatoes.

4. In a small bowl, mix the parsley, orange zest, and garlic. Set aside.

5. Increase the oven temperature to 450°F. Push the vegetables to one side of the dish and add the flounder. Arrange the fish evenly in the pan. Spoon the vegetables over the fish and sprinkle with the parsley mixture.

6. Return the baking dish to the oven and roast until the fish flakes easily with a fork (about 5 minutes for thin fillets and 10 to 12 minutes for thicker fillets). Place the fillets on 4 plates.

Makes 4 servings

Per serving: 302 calories, 24 g protein, 15 g carbohydrates, 16.5 g fat, 2.5 g saturated fat, 54 mg cholesterol, 181 mg sodium, 6 g fiber

Make It a Flat Belly Diet Meal

Serve with ¼ cup steamed brown rice (50)
Total calories: 352

Grilled Salmon Steak

Preparation time: 5 minutes | Marinating time: 30 minutes | Cooking time: 8 minutes

1 tablespoon canola oil
1 tablespoon freshly squeezed lemon juice (about 1 lemon)
Dash ground red pepper
½ teaspoon chopped fresh dill
4 ounces salmon steak

1. In a resealable plastic bag, whisk the oil, lemon juice, pepper, and dill. Add the salmon and massage the bag to coat evenly. Seal and chill for 30 minutes.

2. Preheat a grill to medium. Remove the salmon from the marinade. Pour the marinade into a microwaveable bowl. Cook the salmon for 4 minutes on each side or until opaque. Microwave the marinade on high power for about 2 minutes or until boiling. Drizzle over the salmon.

Makes 1 serving

Per serving: 335 calories, 23 g protein, 1 g carbohydrates, 26.5 g fat, 3.5 g saturated fat, 67 mg cholesterol, 67 mg sodium, 0 g fiber

Make It a Flat Belly Diet Meal

Serve with 2 cups baby greens (15) tossed with 2 tablespoons Newman's Own® Light Balsamic Vinaigrette (45)
Total calories: 395

Lemony Stuffed Sole

Preparation time: 10 minutes | Cooking time: 7 minutes

- 1 pound sole fillets
- ¼ teaspoon salt
- ⅛ teaspoon freshly ground black pepper
- 1 cup Summer Squash Sauté (page 226)
- 1 teaspoon extra virgin olive oil
- ¼ cup dry white wine, or 2 tablespoons freshly squeezed lemon juice mixed with 2 tablespoons vegetable broth
- 1 tablespoon butter
- 2 teaspoons freshly squeezed lemon juice (about 1 lemon)
- ½ teaspoon freshly grated lemon zest
- 1 teaspoon finely chopped fresh parsley
- ½ cup toasted pumpkin seeds

1. Season both sides of the fish with salt and pepper. Place 1 fillet on a flat surface and spread 2 tablespoons of the squash evenly over the top, leaving a ½" margin on both ends. Starting with one end, roll the fillet into a cylinder and secure with toothpick. Repeat with the remaining sole and squash.

2. Heat the oil in 12" nonstick skillet over medium heat and add the fish rolls, seam side up. Cook for 2 minutes. Add the wine or the lemon juice–broth mixture. Reduce the heat to medium low, cover, and cook 5 minutes longer or until the fish flakes easily with a fork.

3. Transfer the fish to a plate and tent loosely with aluminum foil. Add the butter, lemon juice, and lemon zest to the skillet. Remove from the heat, swirl until the butter melts, and spoon over the fish. Remove the picks from the fish and place each roll on a plate. Sprinkle the fish with parsley and pumpkin seeds.

Makes 4 servings

Per serving: 219 calories, 24 g protein, 8 g carbohydrates, 9 g fat, 3 g saturated fat, 62 mg cholesterol, 334 mg sodium, 1 g fiber

Make It a Flat Belly Diet Meal

Serve with 1 cup skin-on cubed roasted red potatoes (100) dressed with 2 tablespoons reduced-fat sour cream (40)

Total calories: 359

Scallop Ceviche

Preparation time: 15 minutes | Chilling time: 1 hour

- ½ **pound bay scallops**
- 3 **tablespoons finely chopped red onion**
- 1 **medium jalapeño chile pepper, seeded and finely chopped (See Note)**
  Juice from 4 limes
- ½ **cup roughly chopped fresh cilantro**
- 1 **small mango, pitted, peeled, and diced**
- ⭐ 1 **cup sliced avocado**

1. In a medium glass bowl, mix scallops, onion, pepper, and lime juice. Cover and chill for at least 1 hour.

2. Remove the scallop mixture from refrigerator. Drain the juice and discard. Mix in the cilantro and mango. Divide the ceviche onto 4 plates. Fan out the avocado slices on the side.

Makes 4 servings

Per serving: 158 calories, 11 g protein, 18 g carbohydrates, 6 g fat, 1 g saturated fat, 19 mg cholesterol, 121 mg sodium, 4 g fiber

Note: Wear plastic gloves and keep hands away from eyes when handling fresh chile peppers.

Make It a Flat Belly Diet Meal

Serve with 1 Thomas'® Whole Wheat Pita (140) and 1 apple (80)
Total calories: 378

Chai Scallops with Bok Choy

Preparation time: 8 minutes | Cooking time: 12 minutes

 2 bags chai tea

2 to 4 heads baby bok choy, quartered lengthwise or halved if small (about ¾ pounds)

 1 tablespoon finely chopped fresh ginger

 1 pound sea scallops, halved horizontally

 ¼ teaspoon salt

 2 teaspoons canola oil

 ⅓ cup light coconut milk

 ½ cup chopped cashews

 1 lime, cut into 4 wedges

1. Bring ½ cup of water to a boil. Remove from the heat and steep the tea bags for 3 minutes. Remove and discard the tea bags. Reserve the brewed tea.

2. Sprinkle the bok choy with ginger. Steam over rapidly boiling water in a covered steamer for about 8 minutes, or until bright green and easily pierced with tip of knife.

3. Pat the scallops dry and sprinkle with salt. Warm the oil in a large skillet over medium-high heat. Add the scallops in a single layer. (Work in batches if necessary.) Cook for 2 minutes on each side or until opaque. Remove from the pan and set aside.

4. Add the tea and coconut milk to the skillet. Cook for 1 to 2 minutes, swirling the pan and allowing the sauce to thicken. Divide the sauce into 4 shallow bowls. Top with the bok choy, scallops, and cashews. Serve with the lime wedges to squeeze over the scallops.

Makes 4 servings

Per serving: 250 calories, 23 g protein, 12 g carbohydrates, 12.5 g fat, 3 g saturated fat, 37 mg cholesterol, 392 mg sodium, 1 g fiber

Make It a Flat Belly Diet Meal
Serve with ½ cup steamed wild rice (150)
Total calories: 400

Sweet and Sour Shrimp

Preparation time: 5 minutes | Cooking time: 6 minutes

- ½ teaspoon olive oil
- 8 ounces frozen stir-fry bell pepper strips
- ⅓ cup apricot jam
- 2 teaspoons red wine vinegar
- 6 ounces (1 cup) cooked, peeled, and deveined shrimp
- ★ ¼ cup chopped unsalted dry-roasted peanuts

1. Heat the oil in a nonstick skillet over medium-high heat. Add the peppers and cook, tossing, for about 3 minutes or until hot. Add the jam and vinegar. Cook for 1 minute or until bubbling. Add the shrimp and cook for 2 minutes or until bubbling. Divide evenly onto 2 plates, sprinkle with the peanuts.

Makes 2 servings

Per serving: 357 calories, 23 g protein, 44 g carbohydrates, 11 g fat, 1.5 g saturated fat, 166 mg cholesterol, 223 mg sodium, 3 g fiber

Make It a Flat Belly Diet Meal
Serve on a bed of 2 cups baby greens (15)
Total calories: 372

Sizzled Shrimp with Heirloom Tomatoes

Preparation: time: 20 minutes | Cooking time: 12 minutes

- 2 teaspoons olive oil, divided
- 1 pound large shrimp, peeled and deveined
- 2 tablespoons finely chopped oil-packed sun-dried tomatoes
- 1 medium red onion, chopped
- 1 cup fresh corn kernels (about 2 medium ears of corn)
- 3 medium heirloom tomatoes, chopped (about 3 cups)
- 4 cloves garlic, minced
- ½ teaspoon salt
- ¼ teaspoon freshly ground black pepper
- ½ cup torn fresh basil leaves
- ½ cup snipped fresh chives
- ⭐ 1 cup sliced avocado

1. Heat 1 teaspoon of the oil in large nonstick skillet over medium-high heat. When hot, add the shrimp and sizzle for 1 minute or until partially cooked. Transfer to small bowl.

2. Add the remaining 1 teaspoon oil to the skillet along with the sun-dried tomatoes, onion, and corn. Cook for 6 minutes, or until the onion and corn are browned. Stir in the tomatoes and garlic. Cook for 3 minutes. Stir in the shrimp and simmer for 1 to 2 minutes, or until the shrimp are opaque.

3. Season with the salt and pepper. Stir in the basil and chives. Spoon the shrimp mixture into 4 shallow bowls. Garnish with the avocado.

Makes 4 servings

Per serving: 248 calories, 22 g protein, 21 g carbohydrates, 10 g fat, 1.5 g saturated fat, 168 mg cholesterol, 515 mg sodium, 6 g fiber

> **Make It a Flat Belly Diet Meal**
>
> Serve with 1 Thomas'® Multigrain Pita (140)
> Total calories: 388

Sesame Seared Scallops

Preparation time: 5 minutes | Cooking time: 10 minutes

16 sea scallops (about 1 pound)

¼ teaspoon kosher salt

2 tablespoons fat-free egg substitute

⅓ cup sesame seeds

1 tablespoon peanut oil

1½ pounds baby bok choy (4 to 6 heads), quartered lengthwise

⭐ ½ cup sunflower seeds

1. Pat the scallops dry and sprinkle both sides with salt. Place the egg substitute in a small bowl. Place the sesame seeds on a small plate. Dip one side of each scallop into the egg substitute and then into sesame seeds. Set aside.

2. Heat the oil in a large skillet over medium heat. Arrange the scallops, sesame side down, with space between them, in the pan. Cook for 3 to 4 minutes, or until the seeds are golden. Flip each scallop carefully without removing the sesame-seed crust. Cook for 6 minutes longer, or until opaque.

3. Meanwhile, put the bok choy into a steamer basket set over a pot of boiling water. Cover and steam for 6 minutes, or until just tender. Nestle the scallops among the bok choy quarters on each of 4 plates. Sprinkle with the sunflower seeds.

Makes 4 servings

Per serving: 280 calories, 20 g protein, 11 g carbohydrates, 19 g fat, 2.5 g saturated fat, 20 mg cholesterol, 345 mg sodium, 5 g fiber

Make It a Flat Belly Diet Meal

Serve with ¼ cup steamed wild rice (75)

Total calories: 355

Thai Sweet-Hot Shrimp

Preparation time: 15 minutes | Marinating time: 30 minutes | Cooking time: 12 minutes

  3 cloves garlic, minced
  1 serrano chile pepper, seeded and minced (See Note)
1½ tablespoons reduced-sodium fish sauce (nam pla) (See Note)
1½ tablespoons sugar
  1 tablespoon freshly squeezed orange juice
  1 tablespoon rice wine vinegar
  ½ teaspoon chile paste
1½ pounds large shrimp, peeled, deveined, and patted dry
  ¾ cup chopped unsalted dry-roasted peanuts

1. In a small saucepan over medium heat, bring first seven ingredients to a boil. Reduce heat to medium and simmer for 3 minutes or until thickened slightly. Remove from the heat and let cool.

2. Place the shrimp in a large bowl. Add 3 tablespoons of the cooled marinade, tossing well to coat. Cover and chill for 30 minutes.

3. Preheat a grill to medium-high. Coat the grill rack with nonstick cooking spray.

4. Thread the shrimp on 6 metal skewers. Grill for 3 to 4 minutes, turning once, until opaque. Divide onto 4 plates, and sprinkle with the peanuts.

Makes 6 servings

Per serving: 230 calories, 25 g protein, 9 g carbohydrates, 11 g fat, 1.5 g saturated fat, 151 mg cholesterol, 375 mg sodium, 2 g fiber

Note: Wear plastic gloves and keep hands away from eyes when handling fresh chile peppers.

Note: Reduced-sodium fish sauce—also called nam pla—can be found in Asian markets.

Make It a Flat Belly Diet Meal

Serve with ½ cup steamed wild rice (150)
Total calories: 380

Seared Wild Salmon with Mango Salsa

Preparation time: 15 minutes | Marinating time: 1 hour | Cooking time: 15 minutes

SALSA

    1 ripe mango, pitted, peeled, and diced (about 1½ cups)
    ½ cup chopped red bell pepper, seeded
    ½ cup chopped red onion
    3 tablespoons freshly squeezed lime juice
    2 tablespoons chopped fresh mint
    1 tablespoon finely chopped jalapeño chile pepper (See Note)
    ¼ teaspoon salt

SALMON

    ¼ cup freshly squeezed lemon juice (about 2 lemons)
    ½ teaspoon paprika
    ¼ teaspoon salt
    2 wild salmon fillets (about 2 pounds, 1" thick)
    1 tablespoon olive oil
  ★ 1½ cups mashed avocado

1. To prepare the salsa: In a small bowl, toss together the mango, bell pepper, onion, lime juice, mint, chile pepper, and salt. Cover and chill at least 1 hour to blend flavors.

2. To prepare the salmon: In a large shallow baking dish, combine the lemon juice, paprika, and salt. Place the salmon in the dish and flip to coat both sides. Marinate, covered, for up to 1 hour in refrigerator.

3. Remove the fillets from the marinade. Discard the marinade. Heat the oil in a large nonstick skillet over medium-high heat. Sear the fillets for 15 minutes, turning once, or until opaque. On each of 6 plates, place ⅓ fillet of salmon topped with ½ cup salsa and ¼ cup avocado.

Makes 6 servings

Per serving: 364 calories, 32 g protein, 15 g carbohydrates, 20.5 g fat, 3 g saturated fat, 83 mg cholesterol, 267 mg sodium, 5 g fiber

Note: Wear plastic gloves and keep hands away from eyes when handling fresh chile peppers.

Flat Belly Diet!

Meat

Dijon Pork Chops with Cabbage

Preparation time: 18 minutes | Cooking time: 36 minutes

- 4 center-cut boneless pork chops (about 1 pound), trimmed
- 4 teaspoons Dijon mustard
- 1 teaspoon plus 1 tablespoon canola oil
- 1 tablespoon grated fresh ginger
- ½ teaspoon ground cinnamon
- ¼ teaspoon ground cloves
- ½ head red cabbage (about 1 pound), cored and shredded
- 2 Granny Smith apples, peeled and grated
- 1 tablespoon pure maple syrup
- ¼ teaspoon salt
- 2 teaspoons cider vinegar
- ½ cup toasted pumpkin seeds

1. Brush both sides of the chops with mustard and set aside. In a large heavy skillet with a lid, warm 1 teaspoon of the oil over medium-low heat. Add the ginger, cinnamon, and cloves. Cook, stirring for 10 to 15 seconds. Add the cabbage, apples, maple syrup, and salt. Stir, reduce the heat to low, cover, and cook for about 30 minutes.

2. Meanwhile, in a heavy skillet heat remaining 1 tablespoon oil over medium-high heat. Arrange chops in a single layer. Cook, flipping halfway through, for about 9 minutes, or until a thermometer inserted in the center of a chop registers 155°F.

3. Add the vinegar to the cabbage mixture. Increase the heat to medium. Cook for about 5 minutes, or until most of the liquid evaporates. Place each chop on a plate with a mound of the cabbage mixture. Sprinkle with 2 tablespoons of the pumpkin seeds.

Makes 4 servings

Per serving: 316 calories, 28 g protein, 25 g carbohydrates, 12.5 g fat, 2.5 g saturated fat, 70 mg cholesterol, 317 mg sodium, 4 g fiber

Make It a Flat Belly Diet Meal
Serve with ¼ cup steamed brown rice (55)
Total calories: 371

Mexican Pork Tenderloin

Preparation time: 10 minutes | Marinating time: 12 hours | Cooking time: 30 minutes

- ½ medium onion, chopped
- 3 cloves garlic, minced
- 2 chipotle chile peppers canned in adobo sauce, finely chopped
- 3 tablespoons cider vinegar
- 2 tablespoons orange juice
- 1 tablespoon sugar
- 2 teaspoons canola oil
- 1 teaspoon chopped fresh oregano
- 1½ pounds pork tenderloin
- ½ teaspoon ground cumin
- ½ teaspoon salt
- ¼ teaspoon freshly ground black pepper
- 1 cup sliced avocado

1. In a small dry skillet, cook the onion and garlic over medium-high heat for 7 minutes. Puree in a blender with the chile peppers, vinegar, orange juice, sugar, oil, and oregano. Place the pork in a shallow dish and cover with paste. Cover and chill overnight.

2. Preheat a grill to medium-high for indirect heat. (If using a charcoal grill, push the coals to one side. If using a gas grill, heat one side to high, the other to medium.)

3. In a small bowl, combine the cumin, salt, and black pepper. Remove the pork from the marinade and blot dry with a paper towel. Rub with the cumin mixture. Grill the pork for 10 minutes. Move to the cooler section of the grill. Cover and grill for 10 minutes more until a thermometer inserted in the center reaches 155°F. Let stand for 10 minutes before slicing. Divide the slices evenly onto 4 plates, top with the avocado.

Makes 4 servings

Per serving: 329 calories, 37 g protein, 11 g carbohydrates, 15 g fat, 3 g saturated fat, 111 mg cholesterol, 416 mg sodium, 3 g fiber

Make It a Flat Belly Diet Meal

Serve with 1 cup grape tomatoes (30)

Total calories: 359

Stir-Fried Rice with Asian Vegetables and Beef

Preparation time 15 minutes | Cooking time 12 minutes

- 1 pouch (10 ounces) frozen brown rice
- 1 sirloin or top round steak (8 ounces, ¾" thick), thinly sliced
- 2 tablespoons reduced-sodium soy sauce, divided
- 2 teaspoons canola oil
- 1 bag (14 ounces) frozen Asian vegetable mix or stir-fry vegetable
- 1 tablespoon finely chopped fresh ginger
- 2 teaspoons finely minced garlic
- ½ cup diagonally sliced scallions
- ½ cup coarsely chopped dry-roasted unsalted peanuts

1. Cook the rice according to the package directions. Set aside.

2. Meanwhile, in a bowl, combine the steak with 1 tablespoon of the soy sauce. Toss to mix. Heat a wok or large skillet over high heat. Add the oil. Place the steak in a single layer and cook without stirring, for 1 minute, to brown. Cook 1 more minute, stirring once or twice, until all the pink in the meat is gone. With a slotted spoon or tongs, transfer the meat to a clean dish and set aside. Add the frozen vegetables to the pan. Cook over medium heat, stirring constantly, for about 5 minutes or until the vegetables are tender.

3. Add the ginger and garlic to the pan and stir-fry for 30 seconds. Add the steak, scallions, peanuts, rice, and the remaining 1 tablespoon soy sauce. Cook, stirring, for about 2 minutes, or until heated through.

Makes 4 servings

Per serving: 330 calories, 21 g protein, 30 g carbohydrates, 15 g fat, 2.5 g saturated fat, 27 mg cholesterol, 356 mg sodium, 5 g fiber

Make It a Flat Belly Diet Meal
Serve with 1 medium orange (70)
Total calories: 400

Vietnamese Beef Salad

Preparation time: 15 minutes | Marinating time: 30 minutes | Cooking time: 8 to 10 minutes

¼ cup reduced-sodium soy sauce

¼ cup freshly squeezed lime juice (about 2 limes)

¼ cup water

2 tablespoons sugar

1 tablespoon minced garlic

2 teaspoons chile paste

½ pound flank steak

6 cups mixed greens

1 cup fresh basil

1 cup fresh cilantro

2 large red onions, thinly sliced (about 1¼ cups)

2 large seedless cucumbers, with peel, julienned

4 medium carrots, julienned

★ ½ cup chopped unsalted dry-roasted peanuts

1. In a medium bowl, whisk together the first six ingredients. Pour 3 tablespoons into a resealable plastic storage bag. Cover and chill the remaining dressing. Add the steak to the bag, seal, and turn to coat. Chill for 30 minutes.

2. Heat a grill or broiler to medium-high heat. Grill the steak for 8 to 10 minutes, turning once, or until a thermometer inserted sideways in the center registers 145°F for medium rare. Let rest 5 minutes and slice thinly at an angle across the grain.

3. In a large bowl, combine the greens, basil, and cilantro. Evenly divide the greens mixture onto 4 plates. Sprinkle on the onions, cucumbers, and carrots. Top each salad with the sliced steak, drizzle with the dressing, sprinkle with peanuts.

Makes 4 servings

Per serving: 323 calories, 22 g protein, 30 g carbohydrates, 14.5 g fat, 3 g saturated fat, 21 mg cholesterol, 654 mg sodium, 8 g fiber

Make It a Flat Belly Diet Meal

Serve with 1 cup red grapes (60)

Total calories: 383

Basic Balsamic Flank Steak

Preparation time: 5 minutes | Marinating time: 1 hour | Cooking time: 16 minutes

- 1 whole flank steak (1½ pounds)
- ⅔ cup balsamic vinegar
- 1 tablespoon black pepper
- 2 cloves garlic
- ¼ cup olive oil

1. Poke the meat with a fork to help the marinade penetrate. Mix the remaining ingredients in a large resealable bag. Drop the steak into the bag, seal, and refrigerate for 1 hour or up to 24 hours.

2. Preheat a grill to medium for direct heat. Remove the meat from the bag, reserving the marinade. Grill the meat for 6 to 8 minutes per side or until a thermometer inserted into the thickest part registers 145°F for medium rare. In a small saucepan, boil the reserved marinade for 5 minutes.

3. Slice the meat diagonally across the grain in thin slices and drizzle with the marinade. Divide evenly onto 4 plates.

Makes 4 servings

Per serving: 393 calories, 37 g protein, 7 g carbohydrates, 23 g fat, 5.5 g saturated fat, 56 mg cholesterol, 108 mg sodium, 0 g fiber

Broccoli and Tofu Stir-Fry with Toasted Almonds

Preparation time: 30 minutes | Cooking time: 12 minutes

- 4 cups broccoli florets
- 1 package (1 pound) extra-firm tofu, diced
- 3 teaspoons toasted sesame oil, divided
- 1 bunch scallions (about 8), trimmed and thinly sliced
- 3 cloves garlic, minced
- 1 small jalapeño chile pepper, seeded and finely chopped (See Note)
- 3½ teaspoons low-sodium soy sauce
- ½ cup lightly toasted sliced almonds
- 2 cups cooked brown rice

1. Lightly steam the broccoli for about 5 minutes, or until crisp-tender. Set aside.

2. Heat 2 teaspoons of the oil in a wok or large nonstick skillet over high heat. When hot, add the tofu and cook, stirring constantly, for 5 minutes or until browned. Transfer to a shallow bowl.

3. Add the remaining 1 teaspoon oil to the wok. Heat for 30 seconds. Add the scallions, garlic, chile pepper, and broccoli. Stir-fry over medium-high heat for 2 minutes. Stir in the soy sauce, almonds, and tofu, tossing gently to combine. Divide the stir-fry and brown rice evenly onto 4 plates.

Makes 4 servings

Per serving: 360 calories, 21 g protein, 33 g carbohydrates, 18 g fat, 2.5 g saturated fat, 0 mg cholesterol, 184 mg sodium, 7 g fiber

Note: Wear plastic gloves and keep hands away from eyes when handling fresh chile peppers.

Make It a Flat Belly Diet Meal
Serve with 1 cup sliced red pepper (40)
Total calories: 400 calories

Quick Chicks

Preparation time: 5 minutes | Cooking time: 18 minutes

- 1 tablespoon olive oil
- ½ medium onion, chopped
- 2 cloves garlic, minced
- 1 teaspoon curry powder
- ½ medium yellow bell pepper, seeded and chopped
- 1 can (28 to 32 ounces) no-salt-added diced tomatoes
- 1 can chickpeas (16 ounces), rinsed and drained
- ½ cup fresh or canned chopped pineapple
- 2 cups thinly sliced fresh spinach
- ⭐ 1 cup mashed avocado

1. Heat the oil in a large nonstick skillet or Dutch oven over medium heat. Add the onion, garlic, and curry powder. Cook, stirring occasionally, for about 3 minutes or until onion starts to soften.

2. Add the bell pepper, tomatoes, chickpeas, and pineapple. Reduce the heat to medium-low and simmer for 10 to 15 minutes or until heated through. Stir in the spinach during the last 5 minutes of cooking. Divide evenly onto 4 plates, top with ¼ cup of avocado.

Makes 4 servings

Per serving: 278 calories, 7 g protein, 35 g carbohydrates, 13 g fat, 2 g saturated fat, 0 mg cholesterol, 319 mg sodium, 10 g fiber

Make It a Flat Belly Diet Meal

Serve with ½ cup cooked Uncle Ben's® Ready Brown Rice (110)
Total calories: 388

Zucchini Rotini

Preparation time: 5 minutes | Cooking time: 10 minutes

- ¼ cup whole wheat rotini pasta, or any other short shape of pasta
- ¾ cup 1% fat cottage cheese
- 1 tablespoon salt-free Italian seasoning
- ½ cup shredded zucchini
- 1 cup canned salt-free diced tomatoes, drained
- ¼ cup reduced-fat shredded mozzarella cheese
- ★ 20 medium black olives, sliced (about ⅔ cup)

1. Prepare the rotini according to the package directions. Drain and set aside.

2. In a microwaveable dish, combine the cottage cheese and Italian seasoning. Stir in the rotini and zucchini. Top with tomatoes and sprinkle with mozzarella. Microwave on high for 3 minutes to warm through. Divide the pasta onto 2 plates, sprinkle on the olives.

Makes 2 servings

Per serving: 223 calories, 18 g protein, 20 g carbohydrates, 8 g fat, 2.5 g saturated fat, 12 mg cholesterol, 864 mg sodium, 4 g fiber

Make It a Flat Belly Diet Meal

Serve with 4 ounces sliced Applegate Farms® Organic Roasted Turkey, rolled up (100) and 1 cup sliced red bell pepper (40)

Total calories: 363

Stewed Vegetables

Preparation time: 10 minutes | Cooking time: 20 minutes

- ¼ cup extra virgin olive oil
- 1 large onion, chopped
- 3 cloves garlic, minced
- 1 can whole tomatoes (16 ounces)
- ½ teaspoon dried thyme
- ⅛ teaspoon salt
- 1 pound green beans, trimmed and cut into 2" pieces
- 1 medium zucchini, halved and sliced
- ½ cup chopped fresh basil

1. Heat the oil in a large nonstick skillet over medium heat. Add the onion and garlic, and cook, stirring occasionally, for 4 minutes or until tender.

2. Add the tomatoes (with juice), thyme, and salt, stirring to break up the tomatoes. Bring to a boil over high heat. Add the green beans. Reduce the heat to low, cover, and simmer, stirring occasionally, for 10 minutes or until the beans are tender.

3. Add the zucchini and cook, stirring occasionally, for 5 minutes or until the zucchini is tender. Remove from the heat and stir in the basil.

Makes 4 servings

Per serving: 194 calories, 4 g protein, 18 g carbohydrates, 14 g fat, 2 g saturated fat, 0 mg cholesterol, 242 mg sodium, 7 g fiber

Make It a Flat Belly Diet Meal

Serve with 3 ounces grilled chicken breast (90) and ¼ cup steamed wild rice (75)

Total calories: 359

Stir-Fried Broccoli and Mushrooms with Tofu

Preparation time: 10 minutes | Cooking time: 8 minutes

⅓ cup chicken or vegetable broth

1 tablespoon apricot all-fruit spread

1 tablespoon reduced-sodium soy sauce

1 tablespoon dry sherry

2 teaspoons cornstarch

1 tablespoon canola oil

1 large head broccoli, cut into florets

4 cloves garlic, minced

1 tablespoon minced fresh ginger

4 ounces fresh mushrooms, sliced

1 cup cherry or yellow pear tomatoes

8 ounces firm tofu, cubed

★ ½ cup toasted chopped cashews

1. In a cup, whisk together first five ingredients. Set aside.

2. Heat the oil in a large nonstick skillet over medium-high heat. Add the broccoli, garlic, and ginger and cook for 1 minute. Add the mushrooms and cook, stirring frequently, for 3 minutes or until the broccoli is crisp-tender.

3. Add the tomatoes and tofu, and cook, stirring frequently, for 2 minutes or until the tomatoes begin to collapse.

4. Stir the cornstarch mixture and add to the skillet. Cook, stirring, for 2 minutes or until the mixture thickens. Divide evenly onto 4 plates and sprinkle with cashews.

Makes 4 servings

Per serving: 283 calories, 16 g protein, 25 g carbohydrates, 16 g fat, 2.5 g saturated fat, 0 mg cholesterol, 246 mg sodium, 6 g dietary fiber

Make It a Flat Belly Diet Meal

Serve with 1 medium orange (70)

Total calories: 353

Spaghetti Squash Casserole

Preparation time: 15 minutes | Cooking time: 7 minutes |
Baking time: 1 hour

- 1 spaghetti squash, halved and seeded
- 1 tablespoon olive oil
- 1 small onion, chopped
- 2 cloves garlic, chopped
- 1 tablespoon chopped fresh basil, or 1 teaspoon dried
- 2 plum tomatoes, chopped
- 1 cup 1% cottage cheese
- ½ cup shredded low-fat mozzarella cheese
- ¼ cup chopped fresh parsley
- ¼ teaspoon salt
- ¼ cup (1 ounce) grated Parmesan cheese
- 3 tablespoons seasoned dry 100% whole grain bread crumbs
- ★ ¾ cup chopped walnuts

1. Preheat the oven to 400°F. Coat a 9" by 13" baking dish and a baking sheet with nonstick cooking spray. Place the squash, cut side down, on the prepared baking sheet. Bake for 30 minutes or until tender. With a fork, scrape the squash strands into a large bowl.

2. Meanwhile, heat the oil in a medium skillet over medium heat. Add the onion, garlic, and basil, and cook for 4 minutes. Add the tomatoes and cook for 3 minutes.

3. Add the cottage cheese, mozzarella, parsley, salt, and the tomato mixture to the bowl with the squash. Toss to coat. Place in the prepared baking dish. Sprinkle evenly with the Parmesan and bread crumbs.

4. Bake for 30 minutes or until hot and bubbly. Sprinkle with walnuts.

Makes 6 servings

Per serving: 254 calories, 13 g protein, 20 g carbohydrates, 15 g fat, 3 g saturated fat, 8 mg cholesterol, 494 mg sodium, 4 g fiber

Make It a Flat Belly Diet Meal

Serve with ⅓ cup canned Alaskan wild salmon (120)
Total calories: 374

Soybeans with Sesame and Scallions

Preparation time: 6 minutes | Cooking time: 14 minutes

- 1 **package (12 ounces) frozen, shelled green soybeans (edamame)**
- 1 **tablespoon soy sauce**
- ½ **cup water**
- ½ **cup slivered almonds**
- 1 **dash hot pepper sauce (optional)**
- 2 **tablespoons minced scallions**
- 1½ **teaspoons toasted sesame oil**
- ⅛ **teaspoon freshly ground black pepper**

1. In a medium saucepan over high heat, bring the soybeans, soy sauce, and water to a boil, stirring occasionally. Reduce the heat to low and simmer for 12 minutes or until tender. If any liquid remains, cook, stirring occasionally, over medium-high heat until the liquid has evaporated.

2. Remove from the heat. Stir in the almonds, hot-pepper sauce (if using), scallions, oil and pepper. Divide onto 4 plates.

Makes 4 servings

Per serving: 212 calories, 13 g protein, 12 g carbohydrates, 13.5 g fat, 1.5 g saturated fat, 0 mg cholesterol, 340 mg sodium, 6 g fiber

Make It a Flat Belly Diet Meal

Serve with ½ cup steamed wild rice (150)

Total calories: 362

Beet and Goat Cheese Salad

Preparation time: 25 minutes

SALAD

- 6 cups baby greens
- 8 medium canned beets (about 8 ounces), drained and sliced
- ⭐ ¾ cup toasted walnut halves

DRESSING

- 2 teaspoons olive oil
- 3 tablespoons white wine vinegar
- ¼ teaspoon salt
  Freshly ground black pepper
- 2 ounces soft goat cheese, crumbled

1. To prepare the salad: Combine the greens, beets, and walnuts in a large bowl.

2. To prepare the dressing: Pour the olive oil into a small bowl, and gradually whisk in the vinegar and salt. Season to taste with pepper. Pour over the salad and toss gently. Portion evenly onto 6 plates, sprinkle on the cheese.

Makes 6 servings

Per serving: 147 calories, 5 g protein, 6 g carbohydrates, 12.5 g fat, 3 g saturated fat, 7 mg cholesterol, 227 mg sodium, 2 g fiber

Make It a Flat Belly Diet Meal

Serve with 1 Thomas'® Multigrain Pita (140) and ¼ cup hummus (100)
Total calories: 387

Balsamic Roasted Carrots

Preparation time: 5 minutes | Cooking time: 25 minutes

8 medium carrots, quartered lengthwise
¼ cup extra virgin olive oil, divided
1 tablespoon balsamic vinegar
½ teaspoon salt
¼ teaspoon freshly ground black pepper

1. Preheat oven to 450°F.

2. In a roasting pan, combine the carrots, 2 tablespoons oil, vinegar, salt, and pepper. Toss to coat. Roast for 20 to 25 minutes, tossing occasionally, until lightly caramelized and tender but still firm. Drizzle with the remaining oil.

Makes 2 servings

Per serving: 232 calories, 2 g protein, 25 g carbohydrates, 14.5 g fat, 2 g saturated fat, 0 mg cholesterol, 752 mg sodium, 7 g fiber

Make It a Flat Belly Diet Meal
Serve with 2 cups organic mixed baby greens (16), 1 cup halved grape tomatoes (30) and 1 Thomas'® Multigrain Pita (140)
Total calories: 418

Mini Sweet Potato Casseroles

Preparation time: 10 minutes | Cooking time: 10 minutes | Baking time: 10 to 12 minutes

- ⭐ ¾ cup finely chopped walnuts
- 2½ tablespoons light butter, melted, divided
- 1½ pounds sweet potatoes, peeled and cut into ½" cubes
- ⅓ cup orange juice
- 2 tablespoons fat-free half-and-half
- ½ teaspoon pumpkin pie spice
- ⅛ teaspoon salt
- ⅛ teaspoon freshly ground black pepper

1. Preheat the oven to 400°F.

2. Set six 4-ounce ramekins on a sturdy baking sheet. Coat the insides of the ramekins with nonstick cooking spray. In a small bowl, combine the walnuts and 1½ tablespoons butter. Mix with a fork to blend. Divide the mixture among the ramekins. Press the walnuts with a fork to cover the bottoms of the ramekins.

3. Place the sweet potatoes in a medium pot and fill with enough cool water to cover potatoes. Bring to a boil. Cover and cook for about 10 minutes or until very tender. Drain, and place the potatoes in a medium mixing bowl. Add the orange juice, half-and-half, pumpkin pie spice, salt, pepper, and the remaining tablespoon of butter. With an electric hand mixer, beat until smooth. Carefully pour the mixture into the ramekins.

4. Bake for 10 to 12 minutes or until lightly browned.

Makes 6 servings

Per serving: 217 calories, 4 g protein, 24 g carbohydrates, 12.5 g fat, 3 g saturated fat, 6 mg cholesterol, 135 mg sodium, 4 g fiber

Make It a Flat Belly Diet Meal

Serve with 4 cups light microwave popcorn (100) and 1 cup sliced red bell pepper (40)

Total calories: 357

Summer Squash Sauté

Preparation time: 10 minutes | Cooking time: 42 minutes

 2 tablespoons extra virgin olive oil

 6 cloves garlic, sliced

 1 teaspoon red pepper flakes

 3 pounds assorted summer squash (such as zucchini, yellow crookneck), thinly sliced into disks

 ½ teaspoon salt

 ★ 1 cup sunflower seeds

1. In a large nonstick skillet set over medium heat, combine the oil, garlic, and pepper flakes. Cook, stirring occasionally, for 2 to 3 minutes, or until the garlic begins to turn golden. Add the squash and salt. Toss to coat. Cover, reduce the heat to medium-low, and cook for 30 minutes, stirring occasionally, until the squash begins to break apart.

2. Uncover the pan and increase the heat to medium. Cook 10 to 12 minutes longer or until the liquid is almost gone. Divide evenly onto 8 plates, sprinkle on the sunflower seeds.

Makes 8 servings

Per serving: 156 calories, 5 g protein, 10 g carbohydrates, 12 g fat, 1.4 g saturated fat, 0 mg cholesterol, 156 mg sodium, 4 g fiber

Make It a Flat Belly Meal

Serve with 4 ounces Applegate Farm Organic Roasted Turkey, rolled up (100), 1 cup red bell pepper sliced (40), and ¼ cup hummus (100)

Total calories: 396

Carrot-Walnut Salad

Preparation time: 20 minutes

⅓ cup golden raisins

2 tablespoons rice wine vinegar

1 tablespoon canola oil

2 teaspoons freshly squeezed lemon juice (about 1 lemon)

1 teaspoon honey

⅛ teaspoon salt

4 large carrots, grated

½ cup toasted chopped walnuts

¼ cup chopped fresh Italian parsley

1. Soak the raisins in hot water for 20 minutes to plump them. Drain.

2. In a small bowl, whisk together the vinegar, oil, lemon juice, honey, and salt.

3. Combine the carrots, walnuts, parsley, raisins, and dressing in a medium bowl and toss to coat. Divide evenly onto 4 salad plates.

Makes 4 servings

Per serving: 199 calories, 3 g protein, 20 g carbohydrates, 13.5 g fat, 1.5 g saturated fat, 0 mg cholesterol, 127 mg sodium, 4 g fiber

Make It a Flat Belly Diet Meal

Serve with 1 slice Food for Life® Ezekiel 4:9® Sesame Sprouted Bread (80) and 1 apple (80)

Total calories: 359

Sugar Snap Pea and Fennel Salad with Apple Cider Vinaigrette

Preparation time: 15 minutes

      2 tablespoons apple cider vinegar
      2 teaspoons honey
  1½ teaspoons extra virgin olive oil
   ¾ teaspoon Dijon mustard
   ¼ teaspoon salt
  2½ cups sugar snap peas, tough strings removed
  1½ cups shelled fresh peas
      1 small fennel bulb, trimmed, halved, and cut into bite-size strips
   ¼ cup grated sweet onion
      1 tablespoon chopped fresh tarragon
      2 teaspoons finely chopped shallots
         Freshly ground black pepper
   ⭐ ¾ cup sunflower seeds

1. Whisk together the vinegar, honey, oil, mustard, and salt in a large bowl. Add the snap peas, peas, fennel, onion, tarragon, and shallot. Toss to coat and season to taste with pepper. Portion onto 6 salad plates, sprinkle on the sunflower seeds.

Makes 6 servings

Per serving: 189 calories, 8 g protein, 19 g carbohydrates, 10.5 g fat, 1 g saturated fat, 0 mg cholesterol, 141 mg sodium, 6 g fiber

Make It a Flat Belly Diet Meal

Serve with ½ cup canned Alaskan wild salmon (180)
Total calories: 369

Wild Rice, Almond, and Cranberry Dressing

Preparation time: 15 minutes | Standing time: 10 Minutes | Cooking time: 1 hour, 15 minutes

- 2 cups wild rice
- 2 strips (½" by 2") orange zest
- 1 rib celery, 3" of leafy top only
- 2 teaspoons salt
- 6 cups water
- 2 whole cloves
- ½ small onion, plus 2 cups chopped onions
- 1 tablespoon olive oil
- 2 cloves garlic, minced
- 2 cups seedless green grapes
- 1 cup unsweetened dried cranberries
- 1 cup fat-free low-sodium chicken broth
- ½ cup chopped flat-leaf parsley
- ⭐ 1 cup toasted sliced almonds

1. In a deep wide 5-quart pot over high heat bring rice, orange zest, celery, salt, and water to a boil. Stick the cloves into the onion half and add to the pot. Cover and cook over medium-low heat for 35 to 45 minutes or until the rice is tender. Remove from the heat and let stand, covered, for 10 minutes. Remove and discard the orange peel, onion with cloves, and celery. Set aside.

2. Heat the oil in a large skillet over medium heat and add the chopped onions. Reduce the heat to low, cover and cook 5 minutes. Increase the heat to medium. Uncover and cook, stirring occasionally, for about 10 minutes. Add the garlic and cook 1 minute. Add the onion mixture, grapes, cranberries, broth, and parsley to the rice and stir to blend. Cover and cook over low heat for 15 minutes. Sprinkle with almonds.

Makes 8 servings

Per serving: 322 calories, 9 g protein, 56 g carbohydrates, 8.5 g fat, 1 g saturated fat, 0 mg cholesterol, 655 mg sodium, 6 g fiber

Make It a Flat Belly Diet Meal
Serve with 1 apple (80)
Total calories: 402

Guilt-Free Fries

Preparation time: 5 minutes | Cooking time: 25 minutes

- 1 large sweet potato and 1 large russet baking potato (1½ pounds total), peeled and sliced into thin strips
- ¼ cup canola oil
- ½ teaspoon chili powder
- ½ teaspoon garlic powder
- ½ teaspoon ground cumin
- ½ teaspoon sea salt

1. Preheat the oven to 450°F.

2. In a bowl, toss together the potatoes, oil, chili powder, garlic powder, and cumin. Arrange the potatoes in a single layer on a baking sheet. Bake for 25 minutes. Halfway through, turn the fries over and continue baking.

3. Remove the fries from the oven and place them on several layers of paper towels. Sprinkle with the salt.

Makes 4 servings

Per serving: 243 calories, 3 g protein, 28 g carbohydrates, 14 g fat, 1 g saturated fat, 0 mg cholesterol, 338 mg sodium, 3 g fiber

Make It a Flat Belly Diet Meal

Serve with 2 cups mixed baby greens (15) and 1 cup halved grape tomatoes (30), tossed with 2 tablespoons Newman's Own® Light Balsamic Vinaigrette (45) and ¾ cup Cascadian Farm® Organic Sweet Corn, thawed (70)
Total calories: 403

Stir-Fried Asparagus with Ginger, Sesame, and Soy

Preparation time: 5 minutes | Cooking time: 12 minutes

1½ pounds asparagus, trimmed and cut into 2″ pieces
¼ cup canola oil
½ large red bell pepper, seeded and cut into strips
1 tablespoon chopped fresh ginger
1 tablespoon reduced-sodium soy sauce
⅛ teaspoon red pepper flakes
2 teaspoons toasted sesame oil
1 teaspoon sesame seeds

1. Bring ¼″ water to a boil in a large nonstick skillet over high heat. Add the asparagus and return to a boil. Reduce the heat to low, cover, and simmer for 5 minutes or until tender-crisp. Drain in a colander and cool briefly under cold running water. Wipe the skillet dry with a paper towel.

2. Heat the canola oil in the same skillet over high heat. Add the bell pepper and cook, stirring constantly, for 3 minutes or until tender-crisp. Add the asparagus, ginger, soy sauce, and pepper flakes and cook for 2 minutes or until heated through. Remove from the heat, and stir in the sesame oil and sesame seeds.

Makes 4 servings

Per serving: 190 calories, 4 g protein, 9 g carbohydrates, 17 g fat, 1.5 g saturated fat, 0 mg cholesterol, 145 mg sodium, 4 g fiber

Make It a Flat Belly Diet Meal

Serve with 4 ounces Applegate Farms® Organic Roasted Turkey, rolled up (100), 1 cup grape tomatoes (30), and 1 medium orange (70)
Total calories: 390

Tuscan White Bean Spread

Preparation time: 10 minutes

- 1 can (15 ounces) cannellini, navy, or great Northern beans, rinsed and drained
- 1 large clove garlic
- 1 tablespoon freshly squeezed lemon juice (about 1 lemon)
- 2 teaspoons white wine vinegar
- 2 sprigs fresh flat-leaf Italian parsley
- 2 basil leaves
- 1 teaspoon Dijon mustard
- $\frac{1}{4}$ teaspoon dried oregano

  Red pepper flakes
- $\frac{3}{4}$ cup olive oil

  Salt

  Freshly ground black pepper

1. In a food processor bowl fitted with a metal blade or in a blender, combine the beans, garlic, lemon juice, vinegar, parsley, basil, mustard, oregano, and pepper flakes to taste. Puree until smooth.

2. With the processor or blender running, slowly pour in the oil until it is all absorbed. Season to taste with salt and black pepper.

Makes 12 servings

Per serving: 140 calories, 1 g protein, 4 g carbohydrates, 13.5 g fat, 2 g saturated fat, 0 mg cholesterol, 87 mg sodium, 1 g fiber

Make It a Flat Belly Diet Meal

Serve with 1 Thomas'® Whole Wheat Pita (140) and 1 cup grape tomatoes (30)

Total calories: 310

Desserts

Plum and Nectarine Trifle

Preparation time: 35 minutes | Standing time: 30 minutes | Chilling time: 1 hour

- 3 plums, pitted and thinly sliced
- 2 nectarines, pitted and thinly sliced
- ¼ cup honey
- 1 tablespoon raspberry or white balsamic vinegar
- 1 cup low-fat vanilla yogurt
- 1 cup part-skim ricotta cheese
- 1 fat-free angel food cake (10 ounces), cut into ½" slices
- ★ ¾ cup toasted slivered almonds

1. In a medium bowl, toss the plums and nectarines with honey and vinegar. Let stand for 30 minutes at room temperature, stirring once or twice.

2. In a small bowl, whisk together the yogurt and ricotta until smooth.

3. Line the bottom of a 2-quart clear glass serving bowl with half of the cake slices. Sprinkle on some of the juice from the fruit. Spread half of the fruit over the cake. Sprinkle on half of the almonds. Spoon on half of the yogurt mixture. Use the remaining cake slices to make a second layer. Top with the remaining fruit. Spoon on the remaining yogurt mixture to cover the fruit. Decorate the top with the remaining almonds.

4. Cover with plastic wrap and chill for 1 hour or up to 24 hours before serving.

Makes 6 servings

Per serving: 371 calories, 13 g protein, 62 g carbohydrates, 10 g fat, 2.5 g saturated fat, 15 mg cholesterol, 289 mg sodium, 4 g fiber

Chocolate Strawberries

Preparation time: 3 minutes | Cooking time: 8 minutes | Cooling time: 30 minutes

⭐ **1 cup semisweet chocolate chips**
1 tablespoon fat-free milk
20 ripe medium strawberries

1. Line a baking sheet with parchment paper.

2. Place the chocolate and milk in the top of a double boiler set over boiling water. Reduce the heat to medium and allow the chocolate to melt, about 3 minutes. Stir until the mixture is smooth. Remove from the heat.

3. Holding by the stem, dip each berry into chocolate, coating three-quarters of the way up. Place on the parchment, leaving 1" of space around each berry.

4. Chill for 30 minutes to set the chocolate.

Makes 4 servings

Per serving: 222 calories, 2 g protein, 31 g carbohydrates, 13 g fat, 7.5 g saturated fat, 0 mg cholesterol, 7 mg sodium, 4 g fiber

Make It a Flat Belly Diet Meal
Serve with 1 cup nonfat cottage cheese (160) sprinkled with cinnamon
Total calories: 382

Pumpkin-Maple Cheesecake

Preparation time: 15 minutes | Cooking time: 1 hour and 10 minutes |
Chilling time: 4 hours

 3 packages (8 ounces each) fat-free cream cheese, at room temperature
²/₃ cup packed brown sugar
 3 large eggs
 1 can (15 ounces) pure pumpkin
½ cup low-fat maple or vanilla yogurt
 2 tablespoons all-purpose flour
1½ teaspoons ground cinnamon
 1 teaspoon ground ginger
 1 teaspoon maple or rum flavoring
 1 teaspoon vanilla extract
⭐ 1½ cups toasted pumpkin seeds

1. Preheat oven to 350°F. With an electric mixer, beat together cream cheese and brown sugar until smooth. Beat in the eggs one at a time. Blend in the pumpkin, yogurt, flour, cinnamon, ginger, maple or rum flavoring, and vanilla extract. Pour the filling into a 9″ springform pan coated with nonstick cooking spray.

2. Bake 1 hour and 10 minutes. Remove from the oven and run a knife around the sides to loosen. Let stand at room temperature for 30 minutes.

3. Chill the cake, uncovered, until cold. Then cover with foil and chill at least 4 hours (or up to 3 days).

4. When ready to serve, carefully remove sides of the pan. Sprinkle each serving with 2 tablespoons of the pumpkin seeds.

Makes 12 servings

Per serving: 299 calories, 20 g protein, 26 g carbohydrates, 13.5 g fat, 3 g saturated fat, 64 mg cholesterol, 315 mg sodium, 2 g fiber

Make It a Flat Belly Diet Meal
Serve with 1 apple (80)
Total calories: 379

Oatmeal Cookies with Cranberries and Chocolate Chips

Preparation time: 10 minutes | Baking time: 10 minutes

> 2 cups rolled oats
> ½ cup whole grain pastry flour
> ¾ teaspoon baking soda
> ½ teaspoon ground cinnamon
> ¼ teaspoon salt
> ½ cup brown sugar
> ⅓ cup canola oil
> 3 large egg whites
> 2 teaspoons vanilla extract
> ¾ cup cranberries, coarsely chopped
> ★ 2¼ cups chopped walnuts
> ½ cup semisweet chocolate chips

1. Preheat the oven to 350°F. In a large bowl, combine the oats, flour, baking soda, cinnamon, and salt.

2. In a medium bowl, whisk together the brown sugar, oil, egg whites, and vanilla extract until smooth. Fold in the cranberries, walnuts, and chocolate chips. Gradually fold in the flour mixture and stir until well blended.

3. Drop the batter by tablespoons onto 2 large baking sheets coated with nonstick cooking spray. Bake for 10 minutes or until the cookies are golden brown.

4. Transfer the cookies to a wire rack to cool completely.

Makes 24 cookies

Per serving (1 cookie): 172 calories, 4 g protein, 15 g carbohydrates, 11.8 g fat, 1.5 g saturated fat, 0 mg cholesterol, 73 mg sodium, 2 g fiber

Make It a Flat Belly Diet Meal

Serve with ½ cup cottage cheese (80) and 1 medium apple (80)

Total calories: 389

Chocolate Pudding with Bananas and Graham Crackers

Preparation time: 5 minutes | Cooking time: 5 minutes | Chilling time: 2 hours

- 3 whole graham crackers, crushed
- 1 ripe banana, sliced
- ½ cup sugar
- ¼ cup unsweetened cocoa powder
- 3 tablespoons cornstarch
  Salt
- 3 cups 2% milk
- ½ teaspoon vanilla extract
- 1½ cups semisweet chocolate chips

1. Evenly divide the graham cracker crumbs among 6 custard cups or ramekins. Press the crumbs to cover the bottom of the ramekins. Top with the banana slices, reserving some for garnish.

2. In a large saucepan, mix the sugar, cocoa, cornstarch, and salt. Stir in the milk. Whisk over medium heat for about 4 minutes or until the pudding comes to a boil and thickens.

3. Cook for 1 minute longer. Remove from the heat and stir in the vanilla extract. Pour into the prepared custard cups. Chill for at least 2 hours, or until set.

4. Sprinkle each custard with ¼ cup chocolate chips and reserved banana slices.

Makes 6 servings

Per serving: 391 calories, 7 g protein, 65 g carbohydrates, 15 g fat, 8.5 g saturated fat, 10 mg cholesterol, 147 mg sodium, 4 g fiber

Citrus Ricotta Cannoli
Preparation time: 15 minutes

  1 container (16 ounces) fat-free ricotta cheese
 ⅓ cup confectioners' sugar
  1 tablespoon freshly grated orange zest
  2 teaspoons freshly grated lemon zest
  1 teaspoon freshly grated lime zest
 ½ teaspoon vanilla extract
  3 cups semisweet chocolate chips, divided
 12 large cannoli shells

1. In a medium bowl, combine the ricotta, confectioners' sugar, orange zest, lemon zest, lime zest, and vanilla extract. With an electric beater, whip until light and fluffy. Gently fold in 2½ cups of the chocolate chips, setting aside the remaining ½ cup.

2. To assemble, spoon the filling into the cannoli shells. Melt the remaining chips and drizzle each cannoli with the melted chocolate.

Makes 12 servings

Per serving (1 cannoli): 250 calories, 6 g protein, 34 g carbohydrates, 13 g fat, 7.7 g saturated fat, 6 mg cholesterol, 42 mg sodium, 3 g fiber

The Four-Week Plan—Journal

Since the Four-Day Anti-Bloat Jumpstart is already under your belt, so to speak, you should already be in the habit of keeping a basic food journal that documents what you eat and how you feel when you're eating it. Recognizing the emotional connection you have with food is critical to losing weight and keeping it off, no matter what plan you're on. But *recognizing* and *fixing* are two different things. During the Jumpstart, I gave you quick Mind Tricks to help you quickly put the focus back on yourself and your goals every time you came in contact with food. You can use these little strategies anytime, anywhere, to put the breaks on "mindless" and emotional eating. But your relationship to food is a lot more complex than what you do and how you feel when you sit down to a meal. Remember the mirror that sent me careening through a fast-food drive-thru? Sometimes, how you feel about yourself and your body can affect how quickly you succumb to that Big Mac® attack.

How to uncover—and unravel—those mysterious connections? Therapy is one way, if you've got the insurance (or cash), and the spare hour every week to spend trying to remember what you ate six days ago and why. Another, more practical way is to maintain a journal. But not just any journal. Most of us have had at least one experience with buying an expensive leather-bound notebook with every intention of capturing our innermost thoughts and feelings, only to find that what we end up with can read like a whole lot of nonsense.

The Flat Belly Diet Journal is different. It isn't a place where you write about the dream you had last night, or the fight you keep having with your husband about why he can't seem to do insert dull but essential household task here. And it's certainly not the place where you brood about your overdemanding boss or underperforming 401(k). The Flat Belly Diet Journal is the place where you explore your relationship to food, where you attempt to dissect the whys and hows of your eating behavior, and where you try to pinpoint the psychological hot buttons that will help propel you to success. (And success in this context means what? Say it with me: a flatter belly!)

I want you to keep this journal with you and use it every single day of this program. Each day, I will give you an exercise in reflection to help you focus your entry. I call these reflections Core Confidences because your confidence level and attitude are at the core of your ability to succeed. There's no need to take all day to complete these exercises. As I assured you in Chapter 6, I would never ask you to do anything I wasn't willing—and able—to do. I certainly can't spend hours a day exploring my relationship to anything. But I can take 15 minutes a day. I can find it on the commuter train or on weekend mornings, just before my girls wake up. If I look for those 15 minutes, I can find them. And so can you.

Core Confidences are essential to forging a true and fruitful mind-belly connection. They will help you discover and understand your motivations, your barriers to success, and the wellsprings of ambition and ability that have driven you to achieve major life goals. It may sound strange, but the same qualities that helped you land a plum job or build a solid relationship with your spouse or raise a healthy, well-adjusted child, are what will help you flatten your belly. Confidence, self-awareness, determination, love, acceptance, compassion, organization—if you have any of these qualities, the Core Confidence exercises will help you tap into and exploit them for your belly's benefit.

Make no mistake: Some of the Core Confidences may not be so fun. Some may ask you to confront difficult personal issues or behaviors you might not be proud of. The Core Confidences will help you uncover your demons, confront them, and fight them.

As you fill out these pages, remember to periodically look back and read what you've written in previous entries. That's how you'll spot behavior patterns, and notice your progress. Each Core Confidence builds upon the last, moving you closer and closer to a deeper sense of self-awareness. Like life itself, it's hard to know where you're going without knowing where you've been.

As with the journal you kept back in Chapter 4, I have three rules for you to follow:

1: Forget spelling and punctuation.

2: Write quickly to ward off your inner critic.

3: Speak from your heart.

Now, let's get writing:

My Flat Belly Diet Journal

Week Number:	Day Number:	Date:

● Core Confidence:

Write down at least three reasons why you have chosen to go on the Flat Belly Diet. Describe how you feel about the 28 days ahead and what you expect from yourself.

_____

_____

_____

_____

_____

_____

_____

_____

● What I Ate Today:

Breakfast: _____ Time: _____

Lunch: _____ Time: _____

Dinner: _____ Time: _____

Snack Pack: _____ Time: _____

● How I Felt Today:

_____

_____

Week Number:	Day Number:	Date:

● Core Confidence:

List four things that will help you succeed on the Flat Belly Diet (example: "my family's cooperation"). Now write about what you are going to do to ensure that you get each of the four things you need.

_____

_____

_____

_____

_____

_____

_____

● **What I Ate Today:**

Breakfast: _____ Time: _____

Lunch: _____ Time: _____

Dinner: _____ Time: _____

Snack Pack: _____ Time: _____

● **How I Felt Today:**

_____

_____

Week Number:	Day Number:	Date:

● Core Confidence:

Practice mindful eating. If you watch TV, check your e-mail, even read the newspaper during meals, you will be distracted from how much and how fast you're eating. Have one meal today in total peace and quiet. Take your time, savor the taste and texture of the food and, eventually, the sensation of fullness. Be conscious of the emotions you feel while you eat. Write about the experience.

_____

_____

_____

_____

_____

_____

● What I Ate Today:

Breakfast: _____ Time: _____

Lunch: _____ Time: _____

Dinner: _____ Time: _____

Snack Pack: _____ Time: _____

● How I Felt Today:

_____

_____

Week Number:	Day Number:	Date:

● **Core Confidence:**

Think of a meal that didn't go well—maybe you overindulged or ate something you later wished you hadn't. Imagine you could go back and "do over" that meal. Write about what you would do differently next time around.

_____

_____

_____

_____

_____

_____

_____

_____

● **What I Ate Today:**

Breakfast: _____ Time: _____

Lunch: _____ Time: _____

Dinner: _____ Time: _____

Snack Pack: _____ Time: _____

● **How I Felt Today:**

_____

_____

Week Number:	Day Number:	Date:

● **Core Confidence:**

Write down two changes you made during the Four-Day Anti-Bloat Jumpstart. How many of these changes turned out to be easier to make than you expected? Describe what happened in each instance.

_____

_____

_____

_____

_____

_____

_____

● **What I Ate Today:**

Breakfast: _____ Time: _____

Lunch: _____ Time: _____

Dinner: _____ Time: _____

Snack Pack: _____ Time: _____

● **How I Felt Today:**

_____

_____

Week Number:	Day Number:	Date:

Core Confidence:

Today, see if you can tell the difference between how it feels to eat when you're feeling hungry and how it feels to eat when you're feeling stressed. Write about those reflections.

_____

_____

_____

_____

_____

_____

_____

What I Ate Today:

Breakfast: _____ Time: _____

Lunch: _____ Time: _____

Dinner: _____ Time: _____

Snack Pack: _____ Time: _____

How I Felt Today:

_____

_____

Week Number:	Day Number:	Date:

● **Core Confidence:**

Today you cross the finish line for Week One. Well done! List the two or three things you found most difficult about being on the Flat Belly Diet. Now write about what you're going to do to clear those hurdles in the week ahead.

_____

_____

_____

_____

_____

_____

_____

● **What I Ate Today:**

Breakfast: _____ Time: _____

Lunch: _____ Time: _____

Dinner: _____ Time: _____

Snack Pack: _____ Time: _____

● **How I Felt Today:**

_____

_____

Week Number:	Day Number:	Date:

● Core Confidence:

Write a personal bio. Who are you, what personal strengths do you bring to your job, family and health Then write a bio on the person you aspire to be. Is she more confident, more active, more compassionate? What qualities can you take from the first to help you become the second?

_____

_____

_____

_____

_____

_____

_____

● What I Ate Today:

Breakfast: _____ Time: _____

Lunch: _____ Time: _____

Dinner: _____ Time: _____

Snack Pack: _____ Time: _____

● How I Felt Today:

_____

_____

Week Number:	Day Number:	Date:

Core Confidence:

Think back over the last few days. Identify one food-related faux pas (maybe you snuck a few Hershey's kisses from the receptionist's desk at work), and write that on the left side of the page. On the opposite side of the page, jot down everything you can think of that you did right that day (made your child laugh, started a project, took a long walk). Now take another look at the 'big picture' of your day. Do you see the one setback in a different light?

_____

_____

_____

_____

_____

_____

_____

What I Ate Today:

Breakfast: _____ Time: _____

Lunch: _____ Time: _____

Dinner: _____ Time: _____

Snack Pack: _____ Time: _____

How I Felt Today:

_____

_____

Week Number:	Day Number:	Date:

● Core Confidence:

Today let's focus on what you're grateful for. Keep listing what you love about your body, your family, your job—even your personal surroundings—until your space is filled.

_____

_____

_____

_____

_____

_____

_____

_____

_____

● What I Ate Today:

Breakfast: _____ Time: _____

Lunch: _____ Time: _____

Dinner: _____ Time: _____

Snack Pack: _____ Time: _____

● How I Felt Today:

_____

_____

Week Number:	Day Number:	Date:

● Core Confidence:

Create a list of five instant indulgences that can be substituted for food when cravings or emotions threaten to get the best of you.

_____

_____

_____

_____

_____

_____

_____

_____

● What I Ate Today:

Breakfast: _____ Time: _____

Lunch: _____ Time: _____

Dinner: _____ Time: _____

Snack Pack: _____ Time: _____

● How I Felt Today:

_____

_____

Week Number:	Day Number:	Date:

Core Confidence:

Write a love note to your belly. Include at least two reasons it deserves your affection and respect.

_____

_____

_____

_____

_____

_____

_____

_____

What I Ate Today:

Breakfast: _____ Time: _____

Lunch: _____ Time: _____

Dinner: _____ Time: _____

Snack Pack: _____ Time: _____

How I Felt Today:

_____

_____

Week Number:	Day Number:	Date:

● Core Confidence:

To learn more about your food/feelings connection, make four columns, labeled **anger, sadness, fear,** *and* **happiness.** *Remember the last couple of times you craved a food when you were experiencing each of those emotions. Think about what you craved—and ate—and note it in the appropriate column.*

_____

_____

_____

_____

_____

_____

_____

● What I Ate Today:

Breakfast: _____ Time: _____

Lunch: _____ Time: _____

Dinner: _____ Time: _____

Snack Pack: _____ Time: _____

● How I Felt Today:

_____

_____

Week Number:	Day Number:	Date:

Core Confidence:

You've just finished Week Two! Congratulations! You're halfway there! Write about how you feel reaching this milestone. Describe the changes you have noticed this week in yourself and your attitudes toward food and your body—your belly in particular. Outline your expectations for the week ahead.

_____

_____

_____

_____

_____

_____

What I Ate Today:

Breakfast: _____ Time: _____

Lunch: _____ Time: _____

Dinner: _____ Time: _____

Snack Pack: _____ Time: _____

How I Felt Today:

_____

_____

Week Number:	Day Number:	Date:

● **Core Confidence:**

Identify three or four "high-risk" scenarios—occasions, activities, or places in which you are in danger of eating more than you should or eating the wrong foods. Now create an escape plan that you can implement to avert trouble in each scenario. Write up a description of this plan, using an "If X, then I'll Y" format.

_____

_____

_____

_____

_____

_____

_____

● **What I Ate Today:**

Breakfast: _____ Time: _____

Lunch: _____ Time: _____

Dinner: _____ Time: _____

Snack Pack: _____ Time: _____

● **How I Felt Today:**

_____

_____

Week Number:	Day Number:	Date:

Core Confidence:

Make a list of at least five activities you've always been interested in but never managed to get around to doing. Rank them in order of preference. Then, alongside each item, enter the very first action you need to take to begin to make it happen.

_____

_____

_____

_____

_____

_____

_____

What I Ate Today:

Breakfast: _____ Time: _____

Lunch: _____ Time: _____

Dinner: _____ Time: _____

Snack Pack: _____ Time: _____

How I Felt Today:

_____

_____

Week Number:	Day Number:	Date:

● Core Confidence:

Plumb your memory banks for unhealthy eating rules you used to follow (like always cleaning your plate). Where did you learn those rules? How do they continue to affect the way you eat? Now write your "New Rules to Eat By" (for example, listen to your stomach and stop eating when it's full).

_____

_____

_____

_____

_____

_____

_____

● What I Ate Today:

Breakfast: _____ Time: _____

Lunch: _____ Time: _____

Dinner: _____ Time: _____

Snack Pack: _____ Time: _____

● How I Felt Today:

_____

_____

Week Number:	Day Number:	Date:

● Core Confidence:

Make a list of all the things and people you're angry with. Then write next to each, in capital letters: I FORGIVE YOU.

_____

_____

_____

_____

_____

_____

_____

_____

● What I Ate Today:

Breakfast: _____ Time: _____

Lunch: _____ Time: _____

Dinner: _____ Time: _____

Snack Pack: _____ Time: _____

● How I Felt Today:

_____

_____

Week Number:	Day Number:	Date:

● Core Confidence:

Try to go through the day appreciating how very much you have. Make a list of five moments you're most grateful for today; read it before you go to sleep.

_____

_____

_____

_____

_____

_____

_____

● What I Ate Today:

Breakfast: _____ Time: _____

Lunch: _____ Time: _____

Dinner: _____ Time: _____

Snack Pack: _____ Time: _____

● How I Felt Today:

_____

_____

Week Number:	Day Number:	Date:

● Core Confidence:

Give yourself a confidence boost. Make a list of all the new things you're doing that you weren't doing three weeks ago. You've probably accomplished a lot more than you think.

_____

_____

_____

_____

_____

_____

_____

_____

● What I Ate Today:

Breakfast: _____ Time: _____

Lunch: _____ Time: _____

Dinner: _____ Time: _____

Snack Pack: _____ Time: _____

● How I Felt Today:

_____

_____

Week Number:	Day Number:	Date:

● Core Confidence:

Welcome to the end of Week Three! Write about how it feels to have come so far. Do you feel empowered? Invincible? Proud? Connected to your belly? Write down all the compliments you've received—including thoughts you've had yourself about how far you've come and how great you look.

_____

_____

_____

_____

_____

_____

_____

● What I Ate Today:

Breakfast: _____ Time: _____

Lunch: _____ Time: _____

Dinner: _____ Time: _____

Snack Pack: _____ Time: _____

● How I Felt Today:

_____

_____

Week Number:	Day Number:	Date:

● **Core Confidence:**

Write today's entry sitting in front of a mirror. Describe who you see as if you were explaining to a friend what this woman looked like. Be as complimentary as possible.

_____

_____

_____

_____

_____

_____

_____

_____

_____

● **What I Ate Today:**

Breakfast: _____ Time: _____

Lunch: _____ Time: _____

Dinner: _____ Time: _____

Snack Pack: _____ Time: _____

● **How I Felt Today:**

_____

_____

Week Number:	Day Number:	Date:

● **Core Confidence:**

If you could have only three foods for the rest of your life, what would they be? Think of a quick recipe—how can you make them fit into the Flat Belly Diet?

_____

_____

_____

_____

_____

_____

_____

_____

● **What I Ate Today:**

Breakfast: _____ Time: _____

Lunch: _____ Time: _____

Dinner: _____ Time: _____

Snack Pack: _____ Time: _____

● **How I Felt Today:**

_____

_____

Week Number:	Day Number:	Date:

● Core Confidence:

In three columns labeled **high, medium,** *and* **low,** *list your motivators in the appropriate column. For example, going down a dress size and being able to walk up a flight of stairs without feeling winded may rank high, while getting a better night's sleep might be a medium.*

_____

_____

_____

_____

_____

_____

_____

_____

● What I Ate Today:

Breakfast: _____ Time: _____

Lunch: _____ Time: _____

Dinner: _____ Time: _____

Snack Pack: _____ Time: _____

● How I Felt Today:

_____

_____

Week Number:	Day Number:	Date:

● **Core Confidence:**

Describe a failure in your recent past. How did you get through it? What was the number-one thing that helped you persevere? How can you apply this to your experience on the Flat Belly Diet?

_____

_____

_____

_____

_____

_____

_____

● **What I Ate Today:**

Breakfast: _____ Time: _____

Lunch: _____ Time: _____

Dinner: _____ Time: _____

Snack Pack: _____ Time: _____

● **How I Felt Today:**

_____

_____

Week Number:	Day Number:	Date:

● **Core Confidence:**

Write about a woman you admire. Why is she so special to you? If you could absorb two of her qualities, what would they be and why?

_____

_____

_____

_____

_____

_____

_____

_____

● **What I Ate Today:**

Breakfast: _____ Time: _____

Lunch: _____ Time: _____

Dinner: _____ Time: _____

Snack Pack: _____ Time: _____

● **How I Felt Today:**

_____

_____

Week Number:	Day Number:	Date:

● **Core Confidence:**

Create a diet motivation booster list: Write down all of the reasons you chose the Flat Belly Diet. Be sure to include what you'll get out of changing that's important to you, both **today** *and in the* **future**. *For example:* **today**—*feel lighter and more energized;* **future**—*not have to take medication. Reread it periodically as a reminder of something you did for yourself.*

_____

_____

_____

_____

_____

_____

● **What I Ate Today:**

Breakfast: _____ Time: _____

Lunch: _____ Time: _____

Dinner: _____ Time: _____

Snack Pack: _____ Time: _____

● **How I Felt Today:**

_____

_____

Week Number:	Day Number:	Date:

● **Core Confidence:**

Congratulations!!!! You've reached the end of the formal Four-Week Plan. Describe how it feels to have set out to complete this program and to actually reach your goal. How healthy do you feel? How happy are you with your results? Write a pledge to yourself that you will continue to fuel your body and your mind in this healthy way.

_____

_____

_____

_____

_____

_____

_____

● **What I Ate Today:**

Breakfast: _____ Time: _____

Lunch: _____ Time: _____

Dinner: _____ Time: _____

Snack Pack: _____ Time: _____

● **How I Felt Today:**

_____

_____

Questions Anyone?

Liz answers some of your most common and pressing queries.

Q: *Why do I have to keep a food journal?*

A: The food journal serves several functions. First, studies show that food journals are incredibly valuable for raising your awareness about exactly what and how much you're eating. Research also tells us that people need accountability, particularly when they're starting out on a new plan, even if it's an accountability to themselves. Writing in a journal each day will help you stay committed to your goals, keep your behaviors on track, and lead you to better results.

Journal in the Digital Age

If you've long ago given up on paper and pens, consider using the journaling feature at **www.flatbellydiet.com**. It allows you to instantly chronicle your relationship to food, *and* easily share your entries with others. This additional feature is key, because Flat Belly Dieters who work together to achieve their goals can be more successful, more focused, and have more fun. Whether or not you choose to share your entries is entirely up to you. You can choose to keep them private, allow certain members or "buddies" to view, or you can share with the entire Flat Belly community. If you choose to share your journal, other members can then comment on your pages, offering support, advice, and encouragement.

www.flatbellydiet.com

The Flat Belly Workout

Three years ago, after I gave birth to Sophia and Olivia, I was anxious (to put it mildly) to get my body back. After nearly two months of doctor-mandated bed rest followed by a Caesarean section, I was desperate to move again. And I planned to do just that. Pre-babies, I had exercised all the time, sometimes devoting 10 to 15 hours a week to working out. I lived in Manhattan, and I'd run five mornings a week, then walk to work, and often take a lunchtime strength training class at the gym. I religiously attended Thursday night yoga classes for years. (As a friend once said, "When you don't have kids, your day can be as long as you want it to be.")

Then the girls came along and I moved to the suburbs. My whole concept of "me" time changed—forever. Once I was back at work, I had way too much to pack into my 9-hour day to squeeze in a lunchtime workout. Mornings were out: I was up at 5:30 a.m. and racing to catch an early train. Yoga classes after work? I dashed out every day at 5:15 to get home in time to spend an hour with my girls before they went to bed. Bottom line: I still needed to exercise, but between an hour-a-day commute, children, and a full-time job, it was simply impossible to keep up my pre-pregnancy schedule.

Clearly, I fully understand how difficult it can be to work exercise into a busy life. That's why it was important to me that the Flat Belly Diet include a workout plan that could be tailored to fit any schedule. Even though this diet plan is designed to provide results if you don't exercise, every expert I know firmly believes in the power of aerobic exercise and strength training to boost your mood and energy levels, and help you prevent disease, maintain bone and muscle mass as you age. Of course, it will also deliver faster results if you're following the Flat Belly Diet, as was demonstrated with our test panelists. Those who added daily exercise lost, on average, 70 percent more body weight and 25 percent more inches than the non-exercisers. While *every single one* of our testers lost fat and inches around their middles—even those who just followed the eating plan—the exercisers lost more, and lost it faster.

The Dynamic Duo: Cardio and Strength

If you're going to exercise, I urge you to do both strength training and aerobic exercise. If you're a walker, try the strength exercises in this chapter. If you're all-weights-all-the-time, then add our suggested aerobic routine to your life. The right mix of cardio and strength exercise is important for fast, lasting results. In one study, women in their 40s did either straight aerobic exercise (60 minutes, 6 days a week) or a mix of workouts (60 minutes of aerobic exercise, 3 days a week, and 60 minutes of strength training, 3 days a week[1]). After 24 weeks, the combo training group lost 40 percent more weight, three times more subcutaneous fat and—here's the kicker—12 percent more dangerous visceral fat. Even better, they also increased lean body mass such as muscle that fuels your metabolism (more on that in a minute).

The Right Reasons to Exercise

Before I get into the workout details, I want to share a few more impressive studies that I'm certain will help bolster your commitment to daily exercise. While diet alone *can* do the trick if you're looking for a flatter belly on this plan, adding exercise will not only speed up your results, it also offers amazing health benefits.

In a study published in the *International Journal of Obesity*, researchers looked at the effect of adding aerobic exercise to a low-calorie diet in overweight and obese women.[2] All followed a reduced-calorie diet, but half of them also included 45 minutes of moderate-intensity step aerobics three times a week and walked for 30 minutes daily. For women who carried more visceral fat than subcutaneous fat, the combo program was 1.3 times more effective than diet alone at shedding belly fat. After 14 weeks, these women lost 40 percent more visceral fat and 57 percent more subcutaneous fat than women who only cut calories. They also reduced their blood pressure 50 percent more and their fasting glucose levels more than twice as much.

Even more remarkable is research from the *Journal of Clinical Endocrinology and Metabolism*.[3] In this study, obese postmenopausal women with type 2 diabetes were split into three groups. One group was given a low-calorie diet high in MUFAs that included a nutrition consultation and

(continued on page 276)

READ A FLAT BELLY
SUCCESS STORY

"I'm not a kid anymore," says 55-year-old Mary Anne Speshok. But you'd never know it from listening to her describe the effect of her new weight loss on her husband of five years. "He's chasing me around the room! Like I'm his toy! He looks at me and says 'Wow! I can't believe what I'm seeing!'"

Mary Ann says her husband is as happy as she is with her results from the first four weeks on the Flat Belly Diet. In just 32 days, she had lost 3½ inches off her hips, 3½ off her stomach, 3 inches off her back—(that little place that hangs over the bra strap), and an inch on each thigh. "On the scale today, I lost 2 more pounds. If feel as if the weight is melting off of me. People tell me I'm walking with more confidence in my step. It's terrific!"

The administrative assistant has a message for anyone considering the Flat Belly Diet: "The only thing you have to do is start it. Don't even think about it. Just start it. All the tools are there."

before   *after*

She calls it a revolutionary, doable winner. Doable, she says, because the MUFAs keep you satisfied. "Most people, including me, don't stay with a diet plan because they get hungry between meals. The difference with this diet is you literally don't get hunger pains. It's revolutionary, because you start seeing results so fast that you want to keep going." And the winner part? "Well," she adds, "just look at what I've lost."

Mary Anne has committed herself to doing the Flat Belly Workout along with the diet. Even though she works full-time and commutes an hour each way to and from work, she still manages to get in her paces. She usually walks 30 minutes at lunchtime, but on days when she can't, she stops in at the gym even before she goes home and does her 30 minutes of walking there. At home, she does either floor exercises or hand weights. She says her energy level is so high these days that exercising is easy.

And like so many recently thin women, Mary Anne has just discovered how great

NOW

it is to fit into a nice, slim pair of jeans. "I never even owned a pair before," she says, adding, "I liked them, but just not on me." Not anymore, though. She says she just went out and bought three different styles of jeans because they all looked so good on her.

In fact, Mary Anne's closet is getting a full workout these days. She's buying new clothes to fit her new body. And she's adding bracelets and necklaces, "which I love. When I felt so big, I just wore my wedding ring and my watch. You don't want to call attention to yourself because you don't feel pretty. But now, bring on the jewelry! The more the better!" She and her husband are renewing their vows soon and she's looking forward to wearing a beautiful gown that she hasn't been able to fit into for a long time. "What a prize for reaching your goal," she exclaims. "To fit into something that sat in your closet, just waiting. This beautiful gown . . . and a size smaller."

Mary Anne has continued to lose! At press time, she was down 34 pounds!

Read Flat Belly Dieters' blogs at www.flatbellydiet.com

www.flatbellydiet.com

weekly support meetings. Another group followed a supervised aerobic exercise program consisting of 50-minute walks, three times a week. The third group received both programs. After 14 weeks, the diet-only and exercise-plus-diet groups lost similar amounts of weight, about 10 pounds, but the combo group lost nearly twice as much visceral belly fat.

A Routine Grounded in Science

When I asked *Prevention*'s fitness director, Michele Stanten, to devise a companion workout plan for the Flat Belly Diet, I knew she'd start by looking for a plan that was backed by the most current research and delivered results. But I had one more request: Our plan had to be easy to follow and work with any schedule. In other words, it had to be something readers could maintain for life. Just like the eating plan, this exercise plan had to be what I call "life-proof." I didn't want any drama attached to it—no running out to buy this or that piece of wacky equipment, no overhauling your basement and turning it into a Pilates studio, no sweating your butt

Did You Know

Cooling down after your workout is just as important as warming up. By slowing your activity and lowering your intensity for 3 to 5 minutes at the end of your workout, you'll transition your body out of exercise mode. (A cool-down is already incorporated into the Flat Belly Diet workouts.) Your heart rate and breathing will come back to normal and blood will be redistributed throughout your body so you finish feeling refreshed instead of dizzy or lightheaded. It also speeds up the removal of lactic acid from the muscles. Feeling good at the end of a workout can improve your odds of getting out there and doing it again tomorrow.

off for months at a time, dreaming of the day you can just lie down in a beach chair and relax already. It had to be a program that most women would find enjoyable, and doable, within the context of their already busy and demanding schedules. Oh, and I had one more directive for Michele: No crunches.

I don't know any woman who loves crunches. All that straining on your neck and lower back, all that huffing and puffing . . . it just doesn't add up. And truth be told, they're not that effective. (In all the research we've seen come out of the exercise labs, the crunch is NEVER the move that is found to target ab muscles the best.) Over the years, I've met top trainers with the most incredibly defined midsections who tell me they moved on from crunches a decade ago. Today, the truly evolved fitness trainers develop belly-centric workouts that don't focus on just one set of ab muscles, but target your whole core—the front, sides, and back.

The Flat Belly Workout Basics

The Flat Belly Workout is built around three main components:

* Aerobic exercise to burn calories, boost cardiovascular fitness, and shed fat

* Strength training with weights to build muscle and boost metabolism

* Core-focused exercises to tone and tighten your midsection.

The first part of the plan, **aerobic exercise**, burns calories, which is the only way to shrink the layer of fat covering your tummy muscles. Unless you're shedding that fat, you can spend hours doing ab exercises without seeing a change. I recommend walking for aerobic exercise because it's easy and accessible and offers loads of benefits, but you can do anything you like: cycling, swimming, jogging, or cardio machines like stair climbers and elliptical trainers. And if you can't fit in all 6 cardio workouts every week, don't beat yourself up: Just do what you can. I want you to customize the workouts so they fit your lifestyle. If you're like me, you'll be much more likely to stick with something that you a) *enjoy* and b) *can actually do*. These days, I'm more about walking and hiking because I can bring my girls along in their stroller (great for my arms too!) rather than the Spinning classes I attended religiously in my 30s. It's all about what works for you, right now, at this point in your life.

In addition to the aerobic workouts, you'll also be doing either the **Metabolism Boost** or the **Belly Routine**. You should aim to do 3 of each weekly. But as I said earlier, if that's not possible, even 1 or 2 of each of these routines a week will help to speed up your results. These workouts are designed to tone and tighten not only your abs, but every inch of your body. So wave good-bye to those jiggly trouble spots on your legs, butt, and arms, along with your belly. The beauty of these strength routines is that each has only 4 or 5 moves—the most effective ones based on research—so you can get firm fast.

NOTE: If you plan to exercise and have to skip one workout, don't skip the metabolism-boosting moves. In the short term, these are the exercises that will translate into higher calorie burning all day long. Plus, as you get older, maintaining and improving muscle becomes essential to preserving lean body mass, protecting your immune system, and maintaining a healthy metabolism.

If you do all 6 workouts one week, make sure to take one **rest day** each week. It doesn't matter what day you choose; feel free to move it around depending on your schedule.

3 Flat Belly Workout Essentials

1) The Cardio Walks

I'm recommending two types of cardio workouts: **Fat Blast** walks and **Calorie Torch** walks. The fat-blasting workout consists of steadily paced walks guaranteed to burn off belly fat. The length of these walks will increase each week, and as you become more fit, you should be able to walk at a faster pace (and burn fat faster!) without feeling any extra effort. The calorie-torching walks are set up to be executed in intervals, meaning periodic bursts of fast-paced walking interspersed with a moderate pace. Studies show that interval training keeps metabolism revved up long after the workout is done. The upshot? You burn more calories throughout the day.

2) The Metabolism Boost

Lifting weights is the single best way to preserve muscle and fuel metabolism. This **Metabolism Boost** workout includes four combo moves that target multiple body parts (like your arms and legs). At the same time, they burn more calories overall and in less time (love that). Each of these moves also has a balance challenge, so while you're working your arms, legs, butt, chest, and back, your core will be constantly engaged. Let me repeat that: *Even while you're doing the metabolism-boosting moves, you will be working the muscles of your belly.*

3) The Belly Routine

This is nothing less than the best and most effective crunch-free exercise routine ever devised. All of the suggested moves have been lab-tested and shown to be up to 80 percent more effective than traditional crunches. And once you've mastered those moves, there's an *advanced* workout using a stability ball to strengthen and tone your midsection even more.

The Benefits of Walking

The way I see it, walking may be the most perfect exercise. It's convenient and inexpensive, with no gyms to join or equipment to buy, other than a good pair of supportive walking or running shoes. In addition to all this are the facts that walking is safe, easy on the joints, can be done absolutely anywhere and at any skill level, and it's beneficial to your health. Have I left anything out?

Oh, yes. It turns out that walking can boost your mood, too. Researchers from Yale University have demonstrated that moderate to vigorous exercise can offset the negative effects of cortisol—the belly-fat-producing stress hormone that we first discussed in Chapter 3.[4] Other research shows that with as little as 10 minutes of exercise, the brain begins to produce endorphins that calm you down and decrease cortisol levels. The mood-boosting benefits of walking begin with the first step you take, carry through to the end of your walk, and last for hours![5]

 Stay Hydrated. Drink at least 2 cups of water about 2 hours before your exercise, and then about 1/2 cup every hour during exercise.

Gear Up for Your Walks

One of the great things about walking is that you don't need any expensive equipment, but there are two very important investments you should make—a good pair of walking shoes and socks. The wrong footwear can cause blisters and injuries and make a normally enjoyable activity a miserable one. So choose them with care.

The Socks

Since some are thick and others are thin, wear your walking socks when you try shoes on because they can affect the fit. Avoid all-cotton socks. Instead look for synthetic fabrics that wick moisture away, keeping your feet dry and making them less prone to blisters.

The Shoes

* **Find a knowledgeable salesperson.** Unlike mass-market retailers, specialty stores often employ trained shoe fitters who will ask you about your walking habits and watch you walk. This information will improve your chances of getting the right shoe for your feet.

* **Get your feet measured.** Your size can change over time, and footwear that's too small can set you up for an array of problems. Make sure you have a thumb's width of room in front of the end of your big toe while you're standing rather than sitting.

* **Replace your shoes every 300 to 500 miles.** That's about every 5 to 8 months if you're walking about 3 miles 5 days a week. By the time a sneaker looks trashed on the outside, the inside support and cushioning are long gone. I know, it's tough to part with a

comfortable pair of old sneakers, but you'll be doing yourself and your feet a favor. Worn-out shoes are a common cause of foot, knee, and even back pain.

The Keys to a Big Calorie Burn: Intensity and Speed

The first thing I need to note is that our walking program is not meant to be a *stroll in the park*. If you want to lose your belly fat, your "walk" must be aerobic enough to get your heart pumping. The program we've set out for you incorporates both *steady paced* and *interval* walks. The steady paced walks are just that. You'll walk at a constant, brisk speed for a certain amount of time, gradually increasing the duration as shown in the plan. And, as you become fitter and your muscles get stronger,

 Walking Outside? Ensure Your Safety

- Walk with a buddy.
- Choose routes you're familiar with.
- Wear reflective clothing and carry a flashlight in the dark and at dawn and dusk. Wear bright colors during the day.
- Try to avoid rush hour to reduce your risk of injury and your exposure to carbon monoxide.
- Don't carry valuables with you.
- Walk facing traffic so you can see cars coming.
- Carry a cell phone and an ID.
- If you listen to music, keep the volume low enough so you can hear if a car or person is approaching you.

Flat Belly Diet!

> **TIP▶** **Avoid heavy meals** During fairly intense activity, as much as 85 percent of blood flow is sent to the muscles, reducing the amount available to your digestive system. Therefore, a too-heavy or hard-to-digest meal before exercise can lead to cramps and competition for blood volume.

you'll naturally walk faster and burn more calories, without it feeling any harder. For instance, a 2-mile walk at 2 mph burns 170 calories (based on a 150-pound person). But when you ratchet it up to 3 mph in that same hour, you'll burn 224 calories—a third more calories, and not an extra minute of exercise time. A win-win situation, don't you agree?

When you do the interval walks, you'll be alternating brisk, paced bouts with faster, higher-intensity bursts. In both cases, you can start with the level that is the most comfortable for you and work your way up as you gain more endurance.

One reason that interval walking works so well is it keeps things interesting. For example, if you're going at a fast pace, within minutes you start to take it down, and just as you think you've got it easy, up it goes to a faster pace again. Even better? Intervals burn more fat than keeping a steady pace. One study followed a group of exercisers who worked out five

> **TIP▶** **Break up your cardio** On days when you're really crunched for time, fit walking into your schedule in other small ways. For example, park your car farther away everywhere you go, take 5 minutes from your lunch break and walk the halls in your office, go inside the bank or coffee shop instead of using the drive-thru, or march in place while you're talking on the phone. Just a few steps here and there can quickly add up throughout the day.

PICK YOUR PACE

Use these pace and exertion levels (based on a 1-to-10 scale) to ensure that you're working out at the right intensity level for your Fat Blast and Calorie Torch Walks.

	HOW IT FEELS	INTENSITY LEVEL	SPEED (MPH) *
WARM-UP, COOL-DOWN	Easy enough that you can sing	3–4	3.0–3.5
BRISK	You can talk freely, but no more singing	5–6	3.5–4.0
FAST	You can talk in brief phrases, but you'd rather not	7–8	4.0+

* Note that these walking speeds are merely guidelines. The fitter you get, the faster you'll walk at each of these levels.

days a week at their target heart rates for up to 45 minutes.[6] They were compared to a group that exercised an identical amount of time but did so in intervals, alternately increasing their intensity 5 beats above their target heart rate and then slowing it down to 5 beats below. After 10 weeks, the group that did the interval training had lost three times as much weight as the first group.

Intensity refers to the level at which you perform your exercise. What is high intensity for someone who has not exercised before may be low

Did You Know

Cardiorespiratory endurance refers to your body's ability to take in and deliver oxygen via your bloodstream to your muscles. The more consistently you exercise, the more your endurance will improve and the easier it becomes to perform aerobic activities like walking or climbing stairs. Before you know it, you'll be able to go longer and faster.

intensity for someone who works out on a regular basis. No matter what your fitness level, you can get a high-intensity workout simply by pushing yourself just a little out of your comfort zone.

Working at high intensity can burn from 25 to 75 percent more calories than exercising at low intensity. Running, biking, even step aerobics all work the same way. The faster you go, or the more effort it takes (say, for example, you're heading up a steep hill), the greater the benefits. You'll be evaluating your level of intensity on a 1 to 10 scale: 1 being how you feel when you're sitting on the couch and 10 being how you'd feel sprinting as fast as you can. For the intensity levels that correspond to the Flat Belly Cardio Walks, see Pick Your Pace, opposite page. It's impossible—and unhealthy—to maintain an extremely high intensity for an entire workout. It's most effective to push yourself into this zone in spurts.

Fat Blast—Steady paced walks to burn off belly fat. Walk at a brisk speed (5–6 intensity level).

Calorie Torch—Interval walks raise your calorie burn during and after your workout to shed even more belly fat. Alternate brisk walking (5–6 intensity level) with short bursts of fast walking (7–8 intensity level).

Get Your Walking Form Up to Speed

The secret to turning your everyday stroll into a fat-blasting stride is proper walking form and technique. The most common mistake people make when they try to pick up the pace is that they take longer strides. This can actually slow you down because your outstretched leg acts like a break, and it can cause injuries due to increased stress on your joints. Instead, take shorter, quicker steps, rolling from heel to toes and pushing off with your toes. Next, bend your arms at about 90-degree angles and

Your Day by Day Walking Schedule

	WEEK 1			WEEK 2		
DAY 1	**FAT BLAST WALK**			**FAT BLAST WALK**		
	TOTAL WORKOUT TIME	HOW IT BREAKS DOWN	INTENSITY LEVEL	TOTAL WORKOUT TIME	HOW IT BREAKS DOWN	INTENSITY LEVEL
	30 minutes	3 min warmup 25 min brisk 2 min cool-down	3–4 5–6 3–4	45 minutes	3 min warmup 40 min brisk 2 min cool-down	3–4 5–6 3–4
DAY 2	**CALORIE TORCH WALK**			**CALORIE TORCH WALK**		
	TOTAL WORKOUT TIME	HOW IT BREAKS DOWN	INTENSITY LEVEL	TOTAL WORKOUT TIME	HOW IT BREAKS DOWN	INTENSITY LEVEL
	25 minutes	3 min warmup 4 min brisk 1 min fast (repeat brisk/fast intervals 4 times) 2 min cool-down	3–4 5–6 7–8 3–4	35 minutes	3 min warmup 4 min brisk 1 min fast (repeat brisk/fast intervals 6 times) 2 min cool-down	3–4 5–6 7–8 3–4
DAY 3	**FAT BLAST WALK**			**FAT BLAST WALK**		
	TOTAL WORKOUT TIME	HOW IT BREAKS DOWN	INTENSITY LEVEL	TOTAL WORKOUT TIME	HOW IT BREAKS DOWN	INTENSITY LEVEL
	30 minutes	3 min warmup 25 min brisk 2 min cool-down	3–4 5–6 3–4	45 minutes	3 min warmup 40 min brisk 2 min cool-down	3–4 5–6 3–4
DAY 4	**CALORIE TORCH WALK**			**CALORIE TORCH WALK**		
	TOTAL WORKOUT TIME	HOW IT BREAKS DOWN	INTENSITY LEVEL	TOTAL WORKOUT TIME	HOW IT BREAKS DOWN	INTENSITY LEVEL
	25 minutes	3 min warmup 4 min brisk 1 min fast (repeat brisk/fast intervals 4 times) 2 min cool-down	3–4 5–6 7–8 3–4	35 minutes	3 min warmup 4 min brisk 1 min fast (repeat brisk/fast intervals 6 times) 2 min cool-down	3–4 5–6 7–8 3–4
DAY 5	**FAT BLAST WALK**			**FAT BLAST WALK**		
	TOTAL WORKOUT TIME	HOW IT BREAKS DOWN	INTENSITY LEVEL	TOTAL WORKOUT TIME	HOW IT BREAKS DOWN	INTENSITY LEVEL
	30 minutes	3 min warmup 25 min brisk 2 min cool-down	3–4 5–6 3–4	45 minutes	3 min warmup 40 min brisk 2 min cool-down	3–4 5–6 3–4
DAY 6	**CALORIE TORCH WALK**			**CALORIE TORCH WALK**		
	TOTAL WORKOUT TIME	HOW IT BREAKS DOWN	INTENSITY LEVEL	TOTAL WORKOUT TIME	HOW IT BREAKS DOWN	INTENSITY LEVEL
	25 minutes	3 min warmup 4 min brisk 1 min fast (repeat brisk/fast intervals 4 times) 2 min cool-down	3–4 5–6 7–8 3–4	35 minutes	3 min warmup 4 min brisk 1 min fast (repeat brisk/fast intervals 6 times) 2 min cool-down	3–4 5–6 7–8 3–4
DAY 7	REST			REST		

FAT BLAST WALK

TOTAL WORKOUT TIME	HOW IT BREAKS DOWN	INTENSITY LEVEL
60 minutes	3 min warmup 55 min brisk 2 min cool-down	3–4 5–6 3–4

CALORIE TORCH WALK

TOTAL WORKOUT TIME	HOW IT BREAKS DOWN	INTENSITY LEVEL
45 minutes	3 min warmup 4 min brisk 1 min fast (do brisk/fast intervals 4 times) 2 min cool-down	3–4 5–6 7–8 3–4

FAT BLAST WALK

TOTAL WORKOUT TIME	HOW IT BREAKS DOWN	INTENSITY LEVEL
60 minutes	3 min warmup 55 min brisk 2 min cool-down	3–4 5–6 3–4

CALORIE TORCH WALK

TOTAL WORKOUT TIME	HOW IT BREAKS DOWN	INTENSITY LEVEL
45 minutes	3 min warmup 4 min brisk 1 min fast (do brisk/fast intervals 4 times) 2 min cool-down	3–4 5–6 7–8 3–4

FAT BLAST WALK

TOTAL WORKOUT TIME	HOW IT BREAKS DOWN	INTENSITY LEVEL
60 minutes	3 min warmup 55 min brisk 2 min cool-down	3–4 5–6 3–4

CALORIE TORCH WALK

TOTAL WORKOUT TIME	HOW IT BREAKS DOWN	INTENSITY LEVEL
45 minutes	3 min warmup 4 min brisk 1 min fast (do brisk/fast intervals 4 times) 2 min cool-down	3–4 5–6 7–8 3–4

REST

FAT BLAST WALK

TOTAL WORKOUT TIME	HOW IT BREAKS DOWN	INTENSITY LEVEL
60 minutes	3 min warmup 55 min brisk 2 min cool-down	3–4 5–6 3–4

CALORIE TORCH WALK

TOTAL WORKOUT TIME	HOW IT BREAKS DOWN	INTENSITY LEVEL
45 minutes	3 min warmup 4 min brisk 1 min fast (do brisk/fast intervals 4 times) 2 min cool-down	3–4 5–6 7–8 3–4

FAT BLAST WALK

TOTAL WORKOUT TIME	HOW IT BREAKS DOWN	INTENSITY LEVEL
60 minutes	3 min warmup 55 min brisk 2 min cool-down	3–4 5–6 3–4

CALORIE TORCH WALK

TOTAL WORKOUT TIME	HOW IT BREAKS DOWN	INTENSITY LEVEL
45 minutes	3 min warmup 4 min brisk 1 min fast (do brisk/fast intervals 4 times) 2 min cool-down	3–4 5–6 7–8 3–4

FAT BLAST WALK

TOTAL WORKOUT TIME	HOW IT BREAKS DOWN	INTENSITY LEVEL
60 minutes	3 min warmup 55 min brisk 2 min cool-down	3–4 5–6 3–4

CALORIE TORCH WALK

TOTAL WORKOUT TIME	HOW IT BREAKS DOWN	INTENSITY LEVEL
45 minutes	3 min warmup 4 min brisk 1 min fast (do brisk/fast intervals 4 times) 2 min cool-down	3–4 5–6 7–8 3–4

REST

swing them forward (no higher than chest height) and back so your hand is almost skimming your hip. Letting your arms flail across your body will slow down your forward momentum. Practice these techniques and you'll be cruising past other walkers in no time.

Strength Training: Muscle in on Belly Fat

I've always been devoted to strength training. (My toddlers know that on Sunday morning, "Mommy goes to make muscles.") It gives me confidence and a sense of empowerment. Plus, I just like the way it makes my body feel: toned, strong, and healthy. I also know how important it is as I get older. Strength training preserves and even rebuilds precious muscle— the body's calorie-burning engine that fuels metabolism. Beginning as early as in your 30s, you start to lose about $\frac{1}{2}$ pound of muscle a year. If you don't take action, that loss can double by the time you hit menopause. With every pound of muscle lost, your body burns fewer calories, which explains why gaining weight gets easier and losing it gets tougher as you get older. Decreasing muscle mass also makes you weaker, and everyday tasks such as getting out of a chair and climbing the stairs become more difficult. As a result, you start to move less—further contributing to muscle loss and fat gain.

Here's how it works: When you challenge a muscle, you create microscopic tears in the muscle tissue. (I know the word " tear" doesn't sound all that healthy, but trust me, in this case it is.) Your body then comes to the rescue and fills those crevices with protein, creating new muscle tissue. This is why you should wait a day between strength training workouts— to give the muscles time to repair themselves.

GREAT RESULTS GUARANTEED: CLIP ON A PEDOMETER

This little device hooks onto your waistband and tracks the number of steps you take throughout the day. As a motivational tool that provides immediate feedback, it's traditionally been used to make getting more exercise easy and fun. Studies show that pedometers can help boost your activity. When a group of 93 women clipped on pedometers, they increased their daily count by 3,788 steps over 8 weeks, according to research published in the *Journal of the American Dietetic Association*.[7]

For the Flat Belly Workout, I recommend that you use a pedometer, but in a slightly different way. One of the reasons some people don't see results when they start an exercise program is because they unconsciously decrease activity in other parts of their day—getting up from their desks less frequently, using the stairs less, or doing fewer activities like chores or walking at a lower intensity level—thereby compensating for their scheduled workouts and negating all or some of the calories burned.

By using a pedometer to get a baseline of your activity level during the Four Day Anti-Bloat Jumpstart in Chapter 4, you can ensure that your everyday activity level doesn't drop off once you start the Flat Belly Workout during Week 1. Here's how it works.

- During the Four-Day Anti-Bloat Jumpstart, clip on your pedometer as soon as you get up in the morning, before you even get out of bed. Then wear it all day long, except in the shower, bath, or pool. When you climb into bed each night, record the number of steps you took. At the end of 4 days, calculate your average daily number of steps by adding each day's total and dividing by 4. This is your daily step goal for the Flat Belly Workout.

- During the four-week Flat Belly Diet, continue to wear your pedometer throughout the day, except when you're doing the prescribed exercises. (These workouts will naturally increase your number of steps, so wearing the pedometer during these sessions will make it difficult to determine if you're slacking off on everyday activities.) Throughout the day, check your step count to make sure you're on track to hit your daily goal. If you're falling behind, increase your activity to ensure that you hit your mark by bedtime.

Replacing the tissue creates stronger muscles—the result you want, because stronger muscle mass makes our bodies look firmer, tighter, and more toned. Most importantly, though, because muscle mass burns about seven times more calories than fat (about 15 more a day per pound), the more muscle you have, the faster you'll burn calories and lose belly fat.

STRETCH YOUR WORKOUT BENEFITS

Stretching after you exercise will increase your flexibility. It will also improve your posture, so you stand taller, making your belly look flatter instantly.

While most of us were taught to stretch before we exercise, the latest research shows no benefits from a pre-workout stretch. The most important thing you can do before exercise is to warm up with gentle activity. If you still want to stretch at the beginning of your workout, do so only after you have warmed up to avoid an injury.

The best time to stretch is post-workout, when your muscles are warm and pliable. This will give you maximum increases in flexibility and range of motion. Stretching then also helps promote recovery.

Here are 5 stretches to target the major muscle groups that you'll be working. Gently ease in and out of the stretches, holding each for 10 seconds. Don't bounce. Do each stretch 3 to 6 times, taking deep breaths throughout.

Chest Stretch

Stand with feet about shoulder-width apart and grasp hands behind back, fingers intertwined and palms facing each other. Keeping chest lifted and shoulders down, squeeze shoulder blades and gently lift arms as high as comfortable. Don't arch back. You should feel a stretch across chest. Hold for 10 seconds and release.

Strength training increases your energy as well, which makes almost every task easier, so you're more likely to remain active throughout the day.

Finally, strong muscles also protects and builds strong bones, which is essential, particularly for a woman. As if losing muscle mass weren't bad enough, women also start to lose bone in their mid-thirties as well, a loss that accelerates as they age, and gathers even more speed going

Back Stretch

Stand with feet about shoulder-width apart. Bending at hips, lean forward and place hands on thighs just above knees. Tuck hips, round back, and drop chin toward chest so back forms a C shape, and you feel a stretch across shoulders and down back. Hold for 10 seconds and release.

Quad Stretch

Standing with feet together, bend left leg behind you, bringing that foot toward buttocks. (You can hold onto a chair or wall with right hand for balance if needed.) Grasp left foot with left hand and tuck hips under so you feel a stretch in the front of left thigh and hip. Hold for 10 seconds and release. Switch legs and repeat.

Calf Stretch

Stand with right foot about 2–3 feet in front of left, toes pointing forward. Place hands on right thigh and bend right knee, keeping left leg straight and pressing left heel into floor so you feel a stretch in left calf. Hold for 10 seconds and release. Switch legs and repeat.

Hamstring Stretch

From the calf stretch position, step back foot in 6 to 12 inches. Straighten front leg, lifting front toes off floor, and bend back leg and sit back, placing hands on thigh. Don't lock front knee. You should feel a stretch down the back of the thigh of your straight leg. Hold for 10 seconds and release. Switch legs and repeat.

Did You Know ?

Stretching itself is not considered a warmup. In fact, to prevent injuries, you should actually warm up before stretching. Doing so helps to improve blood flow to the muscles, making them more pliable and less likely to tear when stretched.

into menopause. At that point, some women begin to lose up to 20 percent of their bone within the first five years. Bone loss can lead to accidental breaks and spontaneous fractures (when bones break for no apparent reason), both of which become harder to heal as we get older, as there is less bone to knit the fracture together. Bone loss also leads to spinal curvature, which, in addition to being uncomfortable, makes standing straight impossible and ultimately causes the belly to protrude. Strength training stresses your bones by stretching and pulling muscles and tendons to increase bone density and reduce the risk of osteoporosis. If you already have osteoporosis, strength training can lessen its impact—but check with your doctor before starting this or any exercise program.

Here are six other ways strength training can improve your health and quality of life:

* You'll sleep better. People who strength train regularly are less likely to struggle with insomnia.

* You'll increase lean muscle mass. Each pound burns about 15 calories per day on its own.

* You'll improve your balance and avoid injury by strengthening ligaments and tendons.

* You'll have more stamina. As you grow stronger, you won't fatigue as easily.

* You'll reduce your diabetes risk. Lean muscle tissue helps your body metabolize blood sugar.

* You'll minimize cellulite. Building firm, compact muscle will smooth out lumpy lower-body fat.

Notes for Strength Training Beginners

If you're not yet doing any strength training, *now is the time to start!* If you're currently lifting weights, then try ramping it up a notch.

The Terms: If you're picking up dumbbells for the first time, here are some strength training basics. The word "rep" is short for *repetition*: for example, each time you lift and lower a dumbbell, or roll your upper body off the floor and then lower it back down, it's considered one repetition. A specific number of reps (8, 10, 12, or so) is called a *set*.

Your Weights: Many women train with weights too light to produce the metabolic boost and body firming they want. Don't be afraid of heavier weights—you won't get big, bulky muscles (women simply don't have enough of the hormones needed for those types of results) but you will get stronger and firmer faster. For the best results, the weight you choose should be heavy enough that by your last rep, you feel like you can't do anymore using good form. If you can, then you need to increase the amount of weight you're lifting. If you can't do at least 8 reps, then the weight is too heavy: Choose a lighter weight or try the easier version of the exercise. Because some muscles are bigger than others, you'll need to use heavier weights for exercises that target your chest, back, legs, and butt.

Did You Know ❓

The fitter you are, the more calories you burn while digesting food. The muscles of women who are active require fuel faster than those of more sedentary women, so their bodies work harder to absorb what they eat. The payoff? More calories burned!

For smaller muscles like your arms and shoulders, you'll probably want lighter weights.

Your Routine: In the Flat Belly Workout, you'll begin with one set of 10 reps and progress up to two sets of 15 reps during the four-week program. Remember, if at any point the weight you're lifting isn't fatiguing the targeted muscles by your last rep, it's time to increase the amount of weight you're using or try the harder variation. (For the ab exercises, you can try the harder version or increase your number of reps.)

Your Equipment: You will need two sets of dumbbells for this section of the program, light and heavy. If you are a beginner, try starting with

5 MINUTES TO BETTER RESULTS

Before you sprint down the street or pick up a 10-pound dumbbell, take 3 to 5 minutes to warm up and prepare your body for activity. By slowly increasing your heart rate, raising your body temperature, and diverting more blood to your working muscles, a warm-up helps you feel better and reduces your risk of injury. Warmups are already included in your walking workouts, and if you do your strength or ab routine right after your walk, you won't need to do any additional warmup. If you're doing the strength or ab workouts separately, march in place for 3 to 5 minutes and simultaneously mimic the exercises that you'll be doing, moving your arms and torso.

a 3-pound and a 5-pound set. If you're more experienced, a 5-pound and 8-pound set it is a good place to begin. Remember, these are general guidelines, so adjust the amount of weight you're lifting based on my recommendations above. Remember, it's easy to determine your correct weight: If the set is so easy that you feel at the end that you can keep going, you're probably not working hard enough—that is, you're not doing enough reps or the weights are too light. If on the other hand, you can barely get the last rep in for the last set, then your choice of weight and pounds is just right. Eventually, as your muscles get stronger, you'll become accustomed to the number of sets and reps you're doing. That's the time to move on.

In the Flat Belly Workout, we give you a specific number of reps to follow, but you can select from our suggestions of how to make it easier or harder depending on what works best for you. Just remember that if you want to develop lean muscle tissue, you must select a weight that's challenging.

A Plan for Metabolism Boosters Only

If you don't want to do the belly firming workout or walk, simply do this routine 3 days a week on nonconsecutive days.

	DAY 2	DAY 4	DAY 6
WEEK 1	The Metabolism Boost 10 reps	The Metabolism Boost 10 reps	The Metabolism Boost 10 reps
WEEK 2	The Metabolism Boost 15 reps	The Metabolism Boost 15 reps	The Metabolism Boost 15 reps
WEEK 3	The Metabolism Boost 2 sets, 10 reps	The Metabolism Boost 2 sets, 10 reps	The Metabolism Boost 2 sets, 10 reps
WEEK 4	The Metabolism Boost 2 sets, 15 reps	The Metabolism Boost 2 sets, 15 reps	The Metabolism Boost 2 sets, 15 reps

Lunge Press

▶ MAIN MOVE

A. Stand with feet together. Holding a dumbbell in each hand, bend arms to 90 degrees so dumbbells are in front of you, forearms parallel to floor, palms facing each other.

B. Step right foot 2 to 3 feet behind you, landing on ball of foot. Bend knees, lowering right knee toward floor until left thigh is parallel to floor. Keep left knee directly over ankle. At the same time, press dumbbells behind you, straightening arms. Hold for a second, then press into left foot, standing back up, bringing feet together, and bending arms back to start position. Do one set, then repeat with opposite leg.

ADAPT IT TO YOUR LEVEL ◀

Make it easier: *Do stationary lunges by starting with left foot 2 to 3 feet in front of right foot, right heel off floor. Maintain this position for one set, then switch legs and repeat.*

Make it harder: *As you stand back up from the lunge position, raise right knee in front of you to hip height, leg bent 90 degrees. At the same time, bend arms back to start position. Hold for one second, balancing on left foot, then swing right foot behind you and repeat. Complete one set, and then repeat with opposite leg.*

Squat Curl

▶ MAIN MOVE

A. Stand with feet together. Holding a dumbbell in each hand, arms down at sides, palms facing forward.

B. Step right foot about 2 feet out to side and bend knees and hips as if you were sitting back into a chair. Sit back as far as possible, keeping knees behind toes. At the same time, bend elbows, curling dumbbells up toward shoulders. Don't move upper arms or shoulders. As you stand back up, bring feet together and lower dumbbells. Complete one set, and then repeat, stepping to side with left foot.

ADAPT IT TO YOUR LEVEL ◀

Make it easier: *Start with feet about shoulder-width apart and maintain this position as you do squats, without stepping to the side.*

Make it harder: *As you stand back up from the squat position, raise left knee, bringing it in front of you to hip height, leg bent 90 degrees. Hold for one second, balancing on right foot, then swing left foot out to side and repeat. Complete one set, then repeat with opposite leg.*

Side Lunge & Raise   The Metabolism Boost

▶ MAIN MOVE

A. Stand with feet together and hold a dumbbell in left hand with arm at side, palm facing in. Place right hand on hip.

B. Step right foot 2 to 3 feet out to side and bend right knee into a lunge, sitting back and bringing dumbbell toward right ankle. Keep right knee behind toes. Press off right foot and stand back up, bringing feet together. From this position, raise left arm out to left side until it's at shoulder height and lift right leg out to opposite side, as high as possible (like photo at right). Hold for a second, then return to start position. Complete one set, then switch sides and repeat.

ADAPT IT TO YOUR LEVEL ◀

Make it easier: *Keep foot on floor as you raise arm to shoulder height.*

Make it harder: *From the lunge position, press off right foot and stand back up, raising left arm out to left side until it's at shoulder height, and lifting right leg out to opposite side, as high as possible, then immediately lower back into another lunge. Complete one set, then switch sides and repeat.*

Pushup Row

▶ MAIN MOVE

A. Holding a dumbbell in each hand, get down on hands and knees. Walk hands forward so body forms a straight line from head to knees, and hands are directly beneath shoulders and feet are in the air.

B. Bend elbows out to sides lowering chest almost to floor. Press into hands, straightening arms back to start position. Then bend right elbow back, pulling dumbbell toward chest, keeping arm close to body. Lower dumbbell back to floor, and repeat from beginning, this time doing a row with left arm. Continue alternating rows for a full set, doing an extra rep each time so you do an equal number of rows with each arm.

ADAPT IT TO YOUR LEVEL ◄

Move 1

Make it easier: *Break up the moves.* **Move 1:** *Do one set of push-ups without dumbbells.* **Move 2:** *Then, get on hands and knees and do a set of rows with each arm.*

Move 2

Make it harder: *Do full push-ups, balancing on hands and toes.*

The Belly Routine

Part 3 of our Flat Belly Workout focuses, of course, on your ab muscles. But I have a confession to make: When I was younger, I often skipped those last 5 minutes of my step class that were devoted to ab exercises for one reason: They consisted solely of crunches. BO-RING. Plus they never seemed to do much for my middle. Our belly-toning workout is a combo routine that includes Pilates, traditional ab moves, and balance exercises to ensure that you're toning your midsection from every angle. All of these moves have been lab-tested and are guaranteed to deliver better results than ordinary crunches.

The roll-up works the main belly muscle, the rectus abdominis, which runs from the bottom of your ribs down to your pelvis, and is 80 percent more effective than a standard crunch.

The bicycle move is our pick if you only have time for one exercise. It targets the main ab muscle more effectively while also getting your obliques, the muscles that wrap around your torso. This generates 190 percent more activity than when you do a simple crunch, according to an American Council on Exercise study.

Did You Know

Sometimes people think they don't have to watch what they eat on the days they've exercised, but this isn't a good practice. People often overestimate the number of calories they burn during physical activity. For example, a 150-pound person burns about 224 calories walking for one hour at 3 miles per hour. That's the number of calories in just one donut, half a muffin, or a 20-ounce bottle of soda. While exercising is always good for your health, splurging on the days you're active can negate some or all of the calories you just worked off and prevent weight loss—or even cause weight gain.

Moves like the plank and arm and leg extension work both ab and back muscles at the same time. Strong back muscles allow you to stand taller, helping your belly look flatter almost instantly.

Finally, the pike zeros in on those lower abs. Since the rectus abdominis is one long, continuous muscle, you can't completely isolate your upper and lower abs. But this exercise allows you to maximize the amount of work that the muscle fibers in the lower portion of that muscle are doing, activating it more than regular crunches, while also stimulating the upper portion.

Bottom line? Not a crunch in the bunch. And now you know why.

A Plan for Belly Firmers Only

If you don't want to do the metabolism moves or walk, simply do this workout 3 times a week on nonconsecutive days.

	DAY 1	DAY 3	DAY 5
WEEK 1	The Belly Routine 10 reps	The Belly Routine 10 reps	The Belly Routine 10 reps
WEEK 2	The Belly Routine 15 reps	The Belly Routine 15 reps	The Belly Routine 15 reps
WEEK 3	The Belly Routine 2 sets, 10 reps	The Belly Routine 2 sets, 10 reps	The Belly Routine 2 sets, 10 reps
WEEK 4	The Belly Routine 2 sets, 15 reps	The Belly Routine 2 sets, 15 reps	The Belly Routine 2 sets, 15 reps

Bicycle

▶ MAIN MOVE

A. Lie face-up with knees above hips, calves parallel to floor, and hands behind head.

B. Contract abs, raising head and shoulders off floor as you extend right leg so it's about 10 inches off floor. Twist to left, bringing right elbow and left knee toward each other. Don't pull on your neck; the work should come from your abs. Hold for a second, then switch sides, twisting to right. That's one rep.

ADAPT IT TO YOUR LEVEL ◀

Make it easier: *Keep feet flat on floor with knees bent as you lift and twist upper body.*

Make it harder: *Lower extended leg farther so it's about 3 inches off floor.*

Hover

▶ MAIN MOVE

A. Lie facedown with upper body propped on forearms and elbows directly beneath shoulders. Toes are tucked.

B. Contract torso muscles, lifting belly and legs off floor so body forms a straight line from head to heels. Keep abs tight so belly doesn't droop. Hold for 15 seconds (increase by 15 seconds each week so that by week 4 you're holding for 1 minute). One rep is all you need to do.

ADAPT IT TO YOUR LEVEL ◀

Make it easier: *Keep knees on floor and just lift belly, balancing on knees and forearms. Stay in this position.*

Make it harder: *Raise right foot off floor and hold for half the time, then switch legs and hold for remaining time.*

Roll-up

▶ MAIN MOVE

A. Lie on back with arms extended overhead and legs bent, feet flat or floor.

B. Inhale and raise arms over chest. Then exhale and roll head toward chest, lifting head and shoulders off floor. (Keep arms next to ears throughout the move.) Press inner thighs together and pull navel in toward spine. Slowly peel off floor until you're sitting up.

C. Then extend legs so you're in a C shape—back rounded, head toward knees, and arms extended in front of you. Gradually reverse the movement, inhaling and squeezing abs as you roll back down to floor, one vertebra at a time.

ADAPT IT TO YOUR LEVEL ◀

Make it easier: *Sit upright on floor with knees bent, feet flat, and arms extended at shoulder height in front of you. As you exhale, roll back about 45 degrees, one vertebra at a time, keeping abs tight. Then roll back up.*

Make it harder: *Do the move with legs extended the entire time.*

Arm & Leg Extension The Belly Routine

▶ MAIN MOVE

A. Kneel with hands directly beneath shoulders, and knees directly beneath hips.

B. Keeping back straight and head in line with spine, simultaneously raise left arm and right leg, extending them in line with back so fingers are pointing straight ahead and toes are pointing back. Hold for a second, then lower. Perform one set, then switch arms and legs and repeat.

ADAPT IT TO YOUR LEVEL ◀

Make it easier: *Instead of lifting and lowering arm and leg, hold them in line with back for 15 seconds, then repeat on opposite side. One rep on each side is enough. Increase the amount of time you hold the move until you can do it for a full minute.*

Make it harder: *When arm and leg are raised, contract abs and draw left elbow and right knee together beneath torso, holding for a second. Extend and repeat. Perform one set, then switch arms and legs and repeat.*

Ab Pike

▶ MAIN MOVE

A. Lie face-up with arms at sides. Bend legs so feet are off floor, thighs over hips.

B. As you pull abs toward spine, lift hips up off floor, keeping legs bent. Keep hands and arms relaxed so you don't use them to help lift. Hold for a second, then slowly lower hips to floor and bend legs.

ADAPT IT TO YOUR LEVEL◀

Make it easier: *Lie with legs bent, feet flat on floor. Contract abs, pressing small of back into floor and curl hips up, doing a pelvic tilt, without lifting feet.*

Make it harder: *As you lift hips, extend legs, and then bend them as you lower.*

Advanced Firming:
A Belly Routine with a Stability Ball

Once you've mastered the basic ab workout, here's a routine using a stability ball to further strengthen and tone your midsection. The principle behind using a large inflatable ball (available at most sporting goods stores) is that it throws off your balance, thus helping you engage and adjust muscles more effectively, which causes your body to sculpt and tone faster. These moves were found by researchers at California State University, Sacramento,[8] to be up to twice as effective as traditional exercises done on the floor when it comes to working ab and back muscles. Follow the same four-week belly schedule as laid out in the chart on page 305.

> **>>> FAST FACT**
>
> According to a study led by researchers at Fred Hutchinson Cancer Research Center in Seattle,[9] getting regular, moderate-intensity exercise may be critically important for postmenopausal women who want to reduce their risk of cancer, heart disease, and other chronic diseases. The reason: Exercise effectively reduces intra-abdominal fat. Even if you exercise regularly but don't see big changes on the scale, you can be confident you're improving your health.

Reverse Hip Lift

▶ MAIN MOVE

A. Lie on back, arms at sides, legs bent, with calves resting on stability ball.

B. Squeeze ball between calves and backs of thighs, contract abs, and lift hips a few inches off floor. Hold for a second, and slowly lower.

ADAPT IT TO YOUR LEVEL ◀

Make it easier: *Place hands under hips.*

Roll Out

▶ MAIN MOVE

A. Kneel with stability ball in front of you at arm's length, and place hands in fists on ball.

B. Keeping abs tight, bend arms as you slowly roll ball away from you so forearms come on ball and body forms a diagonal line from head to knees. Hold for a second, then roll back to start.

ADAPT IT TO YOUR LEVEL ◀

Make it easier: *Bend at hips, keeping them in the air so body forms a tabletop instead of a diagonal plank as you roll forward.*

Pike

▶ MAIN MOVE

A. Balance with thighs on stability ball and hands on floor directly beneath shoulders, body in a straight line from head to feet.

B. Contract abs and lift hips toward ceiling, as if you were going to do a handstand, rolling ball down toward feet.

ADAPT IT TO YOUR LEVEL ◀

Make it easier: *Don't lift hips as high and bend knees, rolling ball to shins.*

Did You Know ⑦

If a 150-pound person walked a dog at a pace of 3 miles per hour for 30 minutes every day, he or she could lose 12 pounds of body fat in one year. Research shows that people who walk with their dogs report they enjoy exercise more, and are more consistent. If you don't have a canine companion, buddy up with a friend or neighbor who does, or volunteer to walk a neighbor's dog.

Skier

▶ MAIN MOVE

A. Balance with shins on stability ball, hands on floor directly beneath, body in a straight line from head to feet.

B. Contract abs, lift hips, and pull knees and ball in toward right arm. Hold then roll out to start position and repeat to left side.

ADAPT IT TO YOUR LEVEL ◀

Make it easier: *Don't bring knees in so far.*

Did You Know

A 3-hour window shopping trip (2 hours of shopping, 1 hour of standing) burns 450 calories. In comparison, 3 hours of watching TV burns less than half that amount.

Put It All Together: Your 28-Day Workout Plan

The Flat Belly Workout is not only optional, but totally customizable. You can do the Walks only, the Metabolism Boost moves only, or the Belly Routine alone. Ideally, as the chart below outlines, you can find the time to do it all.

	DAY 1	DAY 2	DAY 3	
WEEK 1	Fat Blast Walk 30 min	Calorie Torch Walk 25 min	Fat Blast Walk 30 min	
	Belly Routine 10 reps	Metabolism Boost Moves 10 reps	Belly Routine 10 reps	
WEEK 2	Fat Blast Walk 45 min	Calorie Torch Walk 35 min	Fat Blast Walk 45 min	
	Belly Routine 15 reps	Metabolism Boost Moves 15 reps	Belly Routine 15 reps	
WEEK 3	Fat Blast Walk 60 min	Calorie Torch Walk 45 min	Fat Blast Walk 60 min	
	Belly Routine 2 sets, 10 reps	Metabolism Boost Moves 2 sets, 10 reps	Belly Routine 2 sets, 10 reps	
WEEK 4	Fat Blast Walk 60 min	Calorie Torch Walk 45 min	Fat Blast Walk 60 min	
	Belly Routine 2 sets, 15 reps	Metabolism Boost Moves 2 sets, 15 reps	Belly Routine 2 sets, 15 reps	

	DAY 4	DAY 5	DAY 6	DAY 7
	Calorie Torch Walk 25 min	Fat Blast Walk 30 min	Calorie Torch Walk 25 min	REST
	Metabolism Boost Moves 10 reps	Belly Routine 10 reps	Metabolism Boost Moves 10 reps	
	Calorie Torch Walk 35 min	Fat Blast Walk 45 min	Calorie Torch Walk 35 min	REST
	Metabolism Boost Moves 15 reps	Belly Routine 15 reps	Metabolism Boost Moves 15 reps	
	Calorie Torch Walk 45 min	Fat Blast Walk 60 min	Calorie Torch Walk 45 min	REST
	Metabolism Boost Moves 2 sets, 10 reps	Belly Routine 2 sets, 10 reps	Metabolism Boost Moves 2 sets, 10 reps	
	Calorie Rorch Walk 45 min	Fat Blast Walk 60 min	Calorie Torch Walk 45 min	REST
	Metabolism Boost Moves 2 sets, 15 reps	Belly Routine 2 sets, 15 reps	Metabolism Boost moves 2 sets, 15 reps	

Staying Motivated

And now, a word about attitude. By now, you get it. Believing in yourself is integral to this entire Flat Belly journey. I see the power of attitude first-hand in every weight loss success story I edit at *Prevention* magazine, and every time I meet a reader who's faced a life challenge head-on. The right outlook and perspective is what I always call the "special sauce." It means better results, faster results, and results that last.

I urge you to keep this in mind when the going gets rough: Changing your thought process can change your whole workout experience. In fact, your mind is so powerful that it can strengthen muscles without lifting a single dumbbell. When researchers at the Cleveland Clinic had healthy

4 REASONS TO WORK OUT TO MUSIC

1. You'll feel happier A groundbreaking brain imaging study from McGill University showed for the first time that music activates the same reward or pleasure centers in the brain that respond to the good feelings associated with eating and—believe it or not—sex.[10]

2. You'll move faster Australian researchers discovered that the faster the beat, the more vigorously you work out. Other research has shown that exercisers who listen to music have more endurance, and thus exercise longer, burning more calories.

3. You'll get smarter In the first study to look at the combined effects of music and exercise on mental performance, Charles Emery, the study's lead author and a professor of psychology at Ohio State University, found that this duo increased scores on a verbal fluency test.[11]

4. You'll lose belly fat faster Women who exercised to music lost as much as 8 pounds more than women who broke a sweat in silence.

Did You Know (?)

The average person takes about 5,000 steps per day simply going to work, running errands, and doing chores around the house. By taking an extra 5,000 steps, you can decrease body fat and weight, increase "good" HDL cholesterol levels, lower blood pressure, and improve blood sugar levels—all of which help to reduce your risk of heart disease and diabetes.

volunteers imagine that they were contracting the muscles in their hands, they increased hand strength by 35 percent. While this field of study is just beginning, imagine what your mind can do during an actual workout.

Now, armed with this information, head into every workout imagining yourself strong, energized, and light as a feather. Don't recall moments from your tough day or dwell on how tired you feel. Instead, imagine yourself walking on clouds, or that an invisible force is lifting you up, helping you take that next step, lift that weight, or complete that move. Your mind is a powerful thing. Use it! If you take just a few seconds to adjust your attitude, you won't believe how much easier, faster, and enjoyable your workout will be.

Questions Anyone?

Liz answers some of your most common and pressing queries.

Q: *What's the best time of day to exercise?*
A: Some surveys have shown that morning exercisers are more consistent because there are fewer opportunities for you to get sidetracked and skip it than if you do an evening workout. But if you're not a morning person, the snooze button may be all you need to distract you. The most important consideration should be finding a time when you're most willing and able to exercise. Fit your workouts into your life when it's most convenient for you—

otherwise, other activities will always bump exercise off your schedule. There's no significant impact on the calories you burn or how quickly you'll see results based on the time of day you exercise. What matters most is that you *just do it.*

Q: *I understand that exercise is optional on the Flat Belly Diet, but you make a good case for it here. I'm an avid exerciser. Should I stick with my routine or do this routine?*

A: If you have an exercise program you love, absolutely keep it up. You're more likely to stick with exercise if you're doing something you enjoy. But I would encourage you to compare your workouts to those recommended here, and maybe make some minor adjustments to your exercise plan to maximize its belly-flattening potential.

Here are some questions to ask yourself as you review your plan:

✳ *Am I lifting weights at least 2 days a week?*

If not, consider adding the Metabolism Boost moves on pages 296–303 to your workout schedule.

If you are, but want to see better results, aim for 3 days a week of strength training, working in some of the combo moves from the Flat Belly Workout. By working multiple body parts at the same time, you'll burn more calories.

✳ *Am I doing 30 to 60 minutes of cardio exercise (walking, biking, jogging, swimming, cardio machine like an elliptical or stairclimber) at least 5 days a week?*

If not, increase the length or frequency of your workouts to boost your daily calorie burn.

If you are, but want to see better results, turn three of your sessions into interval workouts—like the Calorie Torch walk on page 285. Or, turn any cardio activity into an interval routine by increasing the intensity for 30 to 60 seconds and then slowing down to your usual pace for 2 to 5 minutes. Repeat throughout your workout.

✱ *Am I doing any belly-focused exercises at least 2 days a week?*

If not, start by just doing one or two moves from the Belly Routine on pages 306–315 per session to firm up your midsection.

If you are, but want to see better results, try the Advanced Firming routine on pages 317–323.

Q: *How much did exercise impact the results of your testers?*

A: Adding exercise to the Flat Belly Diet improved results by as much as 70 percent. Our exercise group shed an average of 11 pounds each in 4 weeks—nearly double the non-exercisers, who dropped an average of 6 pounds each (still nothing to sneeze at!). The exercisers also lost 63 percent more inches off their waistlines than non-exercisers, and 25 percent more total inches from head to toe.

But not all the benefits are visible. Exercisers reported improved moods, more energy, better sleep, and a greater sense of confidence. Study after study shows being active lowers your risk of heart disease, diabetes, arthritis, osteoporosis, even cancer—beyond the benefits of eating a healthy diet.

Q: *I'm always famished after I exercise. How can I make sure I don't derail my diet?*

A: The key is timing. You know you shouldn't go more than 4 hours without eating, so you can easily avoid the post-workout munchies by strategically scheduling your workouts in between your meals. By exercising about 3 hours after a meal, you will have allowed enough time for you food to be digested while still being optimally fueled for your workout. And when you're done, it will be almost time for your next meal. In studies where meals were served 15 to 30 minutes after exercise, participants ate less than those who had to wait an hour or more to eat. To ensure you don't fill up on convenience snacks, prepare your Flat Belly Diet meal before you grab your sneakers.

If you still find yourself hungry after exercise, try increasing the amount of water you're drinking before, during, and after your workout. It's possible to mistake thirst for hunger, and water can curb your appetite. People who drink about 7 cups of water a day eat nearly 200 fewer calories than those who get less than a glass a day, reports a study from the University of North Carolina at Chapel Hill.

Your Guide
to Day 33
and Beyond

Here are two revealing statistics: On the one hand, a recent survey found that the percentage of people dieting to lose weight at any given time has fallen to 29 percent, down from 33 percent in 2004.[1] Yet, on the other hand, people are beginning to eat healthier in growing, even stunning, numbers. Fifty-seven percent of shoppers are trying to eat healthfully, up from 45 percent in 2000.[2]

Americans are eating more fruits and vegetables and whole grains than we have in the past, and in some surveys as many as 90 percent are doing something to improve the healthfulness of their meals, like limiting salt, sugar, or saturated fat, or paying more attention to portions. That says to me that people are more interested in making food choices that impact their long-term health than they are in following some gimmicky, quick-fix

READ A FLAT BELLY
SUCCESS STORY

Nicole Michl
Age: 46
Pounds lost: 12 in 32 days
All over inches lost: 11

"I lost 12 pounds in one month plus 3½ inches around the waist and *many* more inches overall! I was thrilled!" exclaims Nicole Michl.

And well she should be. The 46-year-old graphic designer had tried to lose weight off and on over the years, and had even been successful at times. But she could never seem to get rid of her belly fat. "That was always the last to go," she laments. And it was the most annoying to her. So she thought: *If this Flat Belly Diet does what its name says it's going to do—if it's going to help me get rid of my belly fat—I'm going to be one very happy woman.*

Nicole already knew this about herself: When she makes a commitment to something—especially a public commitment—she's more likely to follow it through. So, she challenged herself. "I made the decision to go on the diet—all 32 days' worth—and then I told everyone I knew, so there was no backing out."

before   *after*

She's also the kind of person who, if she commits to something, does it 100 percent. She followed the rules to the letter, she says. "Every single thing they said to do, I did. I bought the right foods. I measured everything. I even followed the diet when I was out, because I know that when you go to a friend's house for dinner, it's so easy to let your guard down—you know, 'I'll try it just this once.' Then, before you know it, you've blown it."

Determined not to let that happen, if Nicole ate at a restaurant, or even if she went away for a weekend, she took along her food in a cooler. "I recently went to a picnic where 50 people sat around eating burgers and other stuff off the grill, and there I was with my little container of food and my bottle of water," she says. "And I looked at what they were eating and what *I* was eating, and I was fine with it. Particularly because so much of what I was eating was organic, and I know that's healthy for me. In fact, I was thrilled with how much of the overall diet is organic."

NOW

Nicole calls the support she had during those 32 days a key to her success. Cheered on the whole way by her family and coworkers, she reveled in her weight loss. "You couldn't help but see the changes in my body," she remarked, "which made me want to keep going. Plus, it was great, knowing they were all in my corner."

Being on the diet slowed her down in what she says is a good way. "I had a tendency to eat really quickly—just to get it over with. Like at work. I know you're not supposed to do this, but I always ate at my desk. When I started the diet, though, I learned to pace myself. I thought about what I was eating and truly appreciated every morsel. Even the portions of nuts. Instead of popping a bunch of nuts in my mouth at once, I'd bite off a piece of one, chew it, and really savor it. I try now to do that with everything." She plans to continue with the diet. With this kind of weight loss *plus* a flatter belly—it's a lifeplan.

Keeping MUFAs in Your Diet

- Choose salad dressings that use olive, canola, or flaxseed oils as a base.
- Have a small handful of nuts and/or seeds for a snack each day.
- Use olive and canola oils for most cooking.

plan. That's why I wanted the Flat Belly Diet to be—first and foremost—something readers could sustain for the rest of their lives.

So, here we are. You've presumably finished the first 32 days of the Flat Belly Diet, so let's take a look back at what you've achieved. If you've followed the parameters of this plan (eating your MUFAs at every meal, limiting calories to 1,600 a day, exercising on a regular basis in a smart, efficient way, and coming to a deeper realization about how you think about food), then you've taken the first and most difficult step toward a healthier future. And—nice bonus here—you've most likely lost a few pounds of the deadliest fat you can have: belly fat.

I also hope you've learned a few things that will make living the Flat Belly Diet lifestyle even more rewarding. You know the anatomy and physiology of the digestive system better than ever before. You understand why the fat you can't see is sometimes scarier than the fat that pokes out over your jeans. And you've read about the intricate connection between stress, cortisol, and your body. Putting all this knowledge to work for you, your belly, and your health in an ongoing way is as simple as permanently adopting the three Flat Belly Diet rules that are probably quite familiar to you by now. I hope you've discovered that it really is possible to follow the Flat Belly Diet forever.

Our test panelists certainly did. After ending the test phase of the Flat Belly Diet, every single one, without being asked, said they planned to stick with the program. Why? Because they lost weight and inches and never felt deprived. Because week after week they reported no hunger, energy through the roof, and no cravings. They gave the meals and recipes rave reviews. And they loved knowing that once they understood the plan, they didn't have to count the days until they could eat satisfying meals again.

Remember, succeeding on the Flat Belly Diet promises an even greater reward than a visually more attractive silhouette: It promises a longer, healthier life. This chapter is all about getting you fully armed to reap *all* the rewards of the Flat Belly Diet—flat belly included—for decades to come.

Flat Belly for Life: Rules to Eat By

* Rule #1 Eat a MUFA at every meal.

* Rule #2 Stick to 400 calories per meal.

* Rule #3 Never go more than 4 hours without eating.

Rule #1: Eat a MUFA at Every Meal

Over the past few weeks, you have come to know MUFAs well (and love them as dearly as I do, I'm sure!), those little miracle workers in your belly that help you feel full *and* lose visceral fat from your middle. You've also discovered how easy—and tasty—it is to include small amounts of these healthy fats in your meals. Even if you can't work in a MUFA at every single meal you ever eat, you know that they are found mainly in vegetable oils, nuts, seeds, olives, and avocados. They are about as easy to come by as they are to love, and it won't be difficult for you to put the MUFA rule into practice most of the time. And if you don't know the MUFA list by heart at this point, you can always flip to page 98 for a quick reference.

Rule #2: Stick to 400 Calories per Meal

I'm not going to mince words here: To keep your weight down and your metabolism on track, you must continue to control your daily caloric intake—that is, stick to about 400 calories per meal, 1,600 per day. Why, you're wondering, do I have to maintain the same daily calorie intake that *got* me to my goal, *after* I've reached that goal? Because the fact of the matter is, 1,600 calories is enough to keep up your energy, support your immune system, and maintain your precious calorie-burning muscle (so you won't feel run down, cranky, or hungry), but it's not enough calories to allow you to gain back your belly fat (and make you more vulnerable to all the attendant health risks).

I am in no way sentencing you to a life of deprivation or boredom here. You've been eating the Flat Belly Diet way for 32 days, and you know firsthand how satisfying and hunger-free this lifestyle is. One of the main reasons the Flat Belly Diet worked for you is that the food is nothing less than fabulous. And there's no shortage of it. And boredom? Forget about it. Between the quick-fix meals, the Snack Packs, and the recipes, as well as a multitude of approved packaged and fast food items, you have hundreds of choices, whether or not you have the time (or the inclination) to cook.

#3. Never Go More Than Four Hours Without Eating

This is your tried-and-true routine by now. You've established a rhythm and your body has responded—by becoming accustomed to having a 3 MUFA-rich 400-calorie meals at four-hour intervals, as well as a healthy Snack Pack at whatever time of day suits you. You now know how it feels to keep your energy up, your blood sugar steady, your metabolism revved—what it's like to have control of your appetite. And you've seen the results, belly-wise. Stick with it and it will continue to benefit your health and your waistline.

DON'T UNDEREAT, EITHER!

It doesn't pay to try to dip below the 1,000-calories-a-day mark. Believe me, I understand the temptation. We've all been led to believe that the fewer calories we ingest, the faster we'll drop the pounds. But weight loss isn't quite that simple. If you drastically cut down on the amount of food you eat for any extended period of time, your body's natural response is to slow things down in order to conserve fat. For those of us who aspire to flatter bellies, that "starvation response" is the last thing we need.

Here's what happens: If you take in too few calories, your body starts breaking down muscle tissue to use for fuel. That muscle loss can drastically affect your metabolism, often for long periods of time. The reason is simple: Muscle is metabolically active tissue that requires a certain number of calories each day to maintain itself, whether or not it's in use. So, the more muscle you have, the more calories you burn. As your muscle mass drops, so does your body's need for calories to sustain it. Let's say a dieter on a too-strict plan loses 15 pounds—10 of which is fat and 5 of which is muscle. Let's also assume that every pound of muscle burns about 50 calories a day. With this muscle tissue gone, the dieter must now consume 250 (5 times 50) fewer calories a day in order to *maintain* her 15-pound weight loss.

Of course, most dieters don't stick with the strict routine for long; they return to their pre-diet eating habits. And that's what puts them at risk of regaining all their lost weight—and then some.

READ A FLAT BELLY
SUCCESS STORY

Evelyn Gomer
Pounds lost: 6
All-over inches lost: 8.5

A lot of Evelyn Gomer's motivation to try the Flat Belly Diet came from her friends—Indirectly, anyway. "For years, I was a city person—New York City, that is. Most city women are skinny and dress beautifully and that was me. For years. Until I moved away from Manhattan." As Evelyn tells it, "I married late in life and moved to the suburbs, where the women were more, well, matronly. So for whatever reason, I just let myself go. Completely." Now, she and her husband have moved back to New York, and she finds her city friends are still skinny and svelte—but she's not. "I wanted to

get back into that," she says. "So when I heard about this diet, I jumped at the chance to try it." It's not that she hadn't dieted before. She had. But not with any lasting success. "This one? What a blessing!"

The first really wonderful thing she found was she was never hungry. "I'm very uncomfortable when I'm hungry.

before　　　*after*

My stomach growls, and I get very tired and listless. But eating the four meals a day worked for me. And those MUFAs!" Like most of the Flat Belly dieters, Evelyn had never heard of a MUFA before being introduced to the diet—at least not by that name—so when she heard she could have nuts, she was happier than happy. "I adore nuts. All kinds. They actually helped alleviate any yen for richer desserts. I still can't believe that something so fattening can be so healthy," she says, adding, "I travel with a jar of peanut butter just in case I'm not in a place where I can find what I want to eat. I can be satisfied just nibbling on nuts. But there are so many other wonderful things to choose from, too."

Evelyn is all about convenience. She read the 28 days of meals and recipes and

NOW

selected about 20 meals that she could be happy with and that didn't require "fifty million ingredients." She's been making those same meals over and over. She says after a while you get to know them by heart and you don't have to read what you need. You do a major shop and you have all the ingredients in the house.

She brings up an additional benefit she has seen from the Flat Belly Diet, one in addition to her 6 pounds and 8 inches lost over four weeks. It seems her husband is getting thinner, too. "No," she says, "He's not on the diet. It's just that I haven't been cooking much, so he's fending for himself and eating a lot less than he usually eats. He's lost weight, and he's very happy about that."

A Flat Belly for Life: Strategies to Live By

Time and again throughout this book I've told you, the Flat Belly Diet is about *attitude*. Well, guess what: so is your healthy, flat-bellied future.

I've supplied you with tools and tricks galore that, as you move forward beyond Day 32, are going to be no less important to nourishing and fortifying yourself than the Flat Belly meals and MUFAs. These tools and tricks have been as integral to your success as the foods you've eaten. You've used them to make major changes. And they'll be just as essential to your ongoing health and well-being.

I've boiled it down to a few key practices and pointers. Use these as a guide for in your journey ahead.

Keep Journaling

As I noted in Chapter 8, journaling is probably the single most important thing you can do going forward to help you maintain your focus on your long-term health goals. Trust me when I say it will help you stay on track. I'm not suggesting that you write something for 15 minutes every day for the rest of your life. I am, however, urging you to keep a journal in your repertoire of health tools. Just as no parent should be without a thermometer in the medicine cabinet, I firmly believe that no woman should be without the means to record her thoughts and feelings on paper (or on a computer). Your journal is your emotional thermometer. Your thoughts are the clues to all your destructive insecurities and all your inner power. Why on earth would you consider ignoring them?

One of the big payoffs from your journal-keeping is that you are well acquainted with many of your vulnerabilities—and the most effective ways to beat them. Being mindful, staying tuned in with yourself, and keeping up with your journaling as much as you can (or even just periodically reading back through your Core Confidence writings) will keep you prepared to handle the inevitable challenges you will encounter in the months and years ahead. If you do take a break from journaling, be sure to complete a Core Confidence exercise when you return. These exercises will keep you focused on the topics at hand: your health and well-being.

Stay Mindful

Whenever you need a quick attitude adjustment from frantic to focused, call on the Mind Tricks from Chapter 4. They're fast—just minutes apiece—but extremely effective at jolting you out of a stress-fueled stupor and adjusting your emotional relationship to eating. They'll help you slow down, take your time, and savor your meals, so you won't be tempted to overindulge or eat too quickly.

Manage Stress

The stress/belly fat connection is clear. Manage stress and you are one step closer to managing your belly fat forever. Writing in your journal can be a great stress reliever, but so can daily exercise. (Another reason that I like to walk to and from work is that I get to work out solutions to office crises in my head, entertaining passersby by occasionally talking to myself.) If you need more ideas to help get your stress under control, peri-

Did You Know

People eat more when they are glued to the television. In a study conducted by Alan Hirsch, MD, neurological director of the Smell and Taste Treatment and Research Foundation in Chicago, 45 volunteers ate as many chips as they wanted while watching late-night talk shows (*The Late Show with David Letterman* and *The Tonight Show* with Jay Leno). The volunteers were also given chips to eat when the television was off. The participants ate an average of 42 to 44 percent more chips while watching TV than when it was turned off. Dr. Hirsch looks to the hypothalamus, home of our "satiety center," for an explanation. If the hypothalamus, which should signal us when we're hungry or full—is distracted (as when watching TV) or "tricked," overeating can result.[3]

odically revisit the stress-busting strategies in Chapter 3 and use as a checklist.

Gather a Support Team

One of the best ways to stay on track and stay motivated is to have a support team behind you. Regardless of how motivated you are, long-term success is always easier with help from others. Even one person will do—just someone to tell you you're doing great every once in a while. Having people in your life who understand and accept your dreams can make all the difference in the world. Your supporters don't have to be members of your family or even good friends, so long as they respect your goals.

Results in the Real World

Scale not budging? At a certain point, every dieter hits a plateau. Here's why it happens. The Flat Belly Diet is designed to only give you enough calories—1,600—to support a healthy, "ideal" weight. If you weigh more than your ideal weight, you are consuming more than 1,600 calories a day. You may jump up and down and tell me that no, you know for a fact that you're only eating 1,200 calories a day, you're starving, and you still don't lose weight. And I would say, *hooey*. Just as you need a certain amount of wood to heat a log cabin, you need a certain amount of calories to keep yourself alive. And the more you weigh, the more calories you need to maintain that weight. Just by going on this plan, you've created a calorie deficit that will allow you to drop pounds. With every pound you lose, however, this calorie deficit shrinks, so as you get closer and closer to your weight goal, it takes longer and longer to lose the next pound.

It doesn't seem fair, but it's the laws of physics! On this plan, you should never hit a true plateau (that is, no net loss). But at times it might feel like your weight loss has stalled. If you're following the plan—and keeping a food journal—I can assure you it has not stalled. It has just slowed. Think about it like this—if you were losing 2 pounds a week, then you're losing just 1 pound a week, you'll eventually get to ½ pound a week, then ¼. Those incremental losses probably won't register on your scale, but a loss is still a loss. Remember that even ¼ pound of fat loss is a full stick of butter zapped from your body. That's still amazing progress in one week's time!

The Flat Belly Diet to Go: The Angst-Free Guide to Dining Out

Okay, you've got this gorgeous, flat belly, you're full of energy, and you feel absolutely wonderful. Now it's time to celebrate. Maybe it's your anniversary. Or your birthday. Or maybe you're just feeling happy. Dinner out? Why not?

Just remember, you are there to celebrate, not binge. And if you stay with the program—or even a slightly modified version—you will wake up feeling good—not guilty—tomorrow. Go ahead, treat yourself to something special. If you plan ahead, there's no reason why you shouldn't be able to enjoy a meal anywhere you want, and that includes pizza with your girlfriends after an afternoon of shopping at the mall.

Following these guidelines will help you stay on track:

* Eat what you would normally eat throughout the day. Skipping a meal in order to save calories for later just increases the chances that you will overeat at dinner. You can also up your exercise—the added calorie burn will help offset a splurge like dessert.

* Have a light snack before you go out. Good options include Flat Belly Diet smoothies or anything that incudes a MUFA. The MUFA will take the edge off your hunger and help you pass up the bread basket.

* Be the first at the table to order. This will keep you from being tempted by others' choices.

* Try to leave some food on your plate. The old "clean plate" rules from childhood no longer apply.

Portion Patrol

Perhaps the most important tip for dining out is to watch the size of your portions. It goes without saying that anything called "super size" is something to be avoided, but beware dishes that don't advertise their generous proportions but provide enough for two or three people. It always helps to have a visual reference to help moderate your portions of different foods when dining out. For example:

* ½ cup of cooked rice or pasta is considered one "serving." This is about the size of a mini fruit cup, or half a baseball. If you're trying to limit your portion of rice or pasta to 2 servings: think 2 mini fruit cups or 1 baseball. Most Chinese restaurants provide far more than this amount of rice.

* One standard sized slice of bread is considered one "serving" of bread. Compare rolls, buns, and other bread products to this mental image and adjust your portion size accordingly: If the bun on your chicken sandwich or burger looks larger than 2 slices of bread, leave some bread on the plate.

* 3 ounces of cooked meat, the size of a deck of cards or woman's palm, is considered one "serving." Most restaurants provide far

more than this amount in an entrée. Savvy ways to cut back include ordering a half portion, a sandwich instead of an entrée, or splitting a meal.

* ¼ cup of shredded cheese is considered a single portion. That's about the size of a golf ball. According to the 2005 Dietary Guidelines, healthy adults need 2 to 3 servings of milk, yogurt, or cheese per day. If cheese is your weakness, think "golf ball" the next time you sprinkle cheese on your food.

In Closing

I'd like to close by reminding you of the very last question I asked you in Chapter 3: *Who are you doing this for?* There is still only one acceptable answer to that question, whether you choose to continue with this plan one day at a time, or enroll in the online service **flatbellydiet.com** for life. That answer is you. If you weren't quite sure of that back then, I hope that I have given you the tools to arrive at that answer now.

The Core Confidences in Chapter 8 were devised to help you arrive at that answer, and this plan as a whole was created to help you see that focusing on yourself isn't an exercise in selfishness. In today's day and age, we are all overly committed to other people, whether it's the attention we lavish on our children and spouse, or the time we spend at our jobs, or the effort we put into building our communities. But I speak from experience when I tell you that none of those commitments is worth anything if you aren't first and foremost committed to yourself. The Flat Belly Diet is not a vanity ploy. Sure, it's a weight-loss plan designed to give you a sexier waistline. But it's not a crazy detox diet that promises you the abs of a 20-year-old. It is a weight-loss plan based on the most credible—and safe—

science that targets the most dangerous type of fat you carry on your body, the fat that threatens your very existence. If you want to live longer and healthier, keeping that fat is simply not an option.

I hope that you will continue to eat the Flat Belly Diet way for as long as it takes for you to experience the freedom that comes from a healthier body weight. If you end up with the abs of steel, I will be over-the-moon thrilled for you! (Although maybe just a teensy bit jealous.) But I'd be just as happy if you were to tell me that you lost your pregnancy weight, or you started walking, or you finally stopped buying shapeless, oversized tunics because you no longer feel self-conscious about the way you look. This plan is less about achieving an ideal body than it is about creating a healthier life. If you remember nothing about the Flat Belly Diet but the fact that a MUFA at every meal could save your life, then I've done my job. And you've done yours.

End Notes

Chapter 1

1. J.A. Paniagua, A. Gallego de la Sacristana, I. Romero, A. Vidal-Puig, J.M. Latre, E. Sanchez, P. Perez-Martinez, J. Lopez-Miranda, and F. Perez-Jimenez, "Monounsaturated Fat–Rich Diet Prevents Central Body Fat Distribution and Decreases Postprandial Adiponectin Expression Induced by a Carbohydrate-Rich Diet in Insulin-Resistant Subjects," *Diabetes Care* 30 (2007): 1717–23.

Chapter 2

1. "Tendency to Overeat During the Holidays Can Be Traced to Ancestors," interview with Vaughn Bryant, PhD, *Texas A&M News,* December 2006, http://tamunews.tamu.edu/archives/article.php?articleid=3884&month=12&year2006.
2. Renee Cree, Temple University, "Food Choices When Eating Out Affect BMI," *Medical News Today,* October 23, 2007, www.medicalnewstoday.com/articles/86361.php.
3. Frank B. Hu; Tricia Y. Li; Graham A. Colditz; Walter C. Willett; JoAnn E. Manson, "Television Watching and Other Sedentary Behaviors in Relation to Risk of Obesity and Type 2 Diabetes Mellitus in Women," *JAMA,* 289 (2003):1785–91.
4. R.E. Ostlund, M. Staten, W.M. Kohrt, J. Schultz, and M. Malley, "The Ratio of Waist-to-Hip Circumference, Plasma Insulin Level, and Glucose Intolerance as Independent Predictors of the HDL2 Cholesterol Level in Older Adults," *New England Journal of Medicine,* 322, no. 4 (January 25, 1990):229–34.
5. László B. Tankó, Yu Z. Bagger, Peter Alexandersen, Philip J. Larsen, Claus Christiansen, "Peripheral Adiposity Exhibits an Independent Dominant Antiatherogenic Effect in Elderly Women," *Circulation,*107 (2003):1626.

6. R.A. Whitmer, S. Sidney, J. Selby, S. Claiborne Johnston, and K. Yaffe, "Midlife Cardiovascular Risk Factors and Risk of Dementia in Late Life," *Neurology*, 64 (2005):277–81.

7. Salim Yusuf, Steven Hawken, et al. "Obesity and the Risk of Myocardial Infarction in 27,000 Participants from 52 Countries; A Case-Control Study," *Lancet*, 366 (2005):1640–49.

8. http://win.niddk.nih.gov/publications/tools.htm#circumf.

9. http://www.rush.edu/itools/hip/hipcalc.html.

10. "Modest Gain in Visceral Fat Causes Dysfunction of Blood Vessel Lining in Lean Healthy Humans; Shedding Weight Restores Vessel Health," presented by the Mayo Clinic team at the American Heart Association's Scientific Sessions, November 2007, http://www.sciencedaily.com/releases/2007/11/071105121934.htm

11. "Thin People May Be Obese on the Inside," *Medical Research News,* May 14,2007, reporting a study funded by the Medical Research Council under the direction of Dr. Jimmy Bell, Professor of Molecular Imaging at Imperial College, London, http://www.news-medical.net/?id=25076.

Chapter 3

1. Doreen Virtue, *Constant Craving A–Z* (Carlsbad, CA: Hay House, 1999).

2. Jennifer A. Linde, Robert W. Jeffery, Simone A. French, Nicolaas P. Pronk, Raymond G. Boyle, "Self-Weighing in Weight Gain Prevention and Weight Loss Trials," *Annals of Behavioral Medicine,* 30, no. 3 (2005): 210–16.

3. http://www.foodandmood.org/Pages/sh-survey.html

4. Jos A. Bosch, Eco J.C. de Geus, Angele Kelder, Enno C.I. Veerman, Johan Hoogstraten, and Arie V. Nieuw Amerongen, "Differential Effects of Active versus Passive Coping on Secretory Immunity," *Psychophysiology,* 38, no. 5 (2001), doi:10.1111/1469-8986.3850836.

5. Mikko Laaksonen, Sirpa Sarlio-Lähteenkorva, Päivi Leino-Arjas, Pekka Martikainen, and Eero Lahelma, "Body Weight and Health Status: Importance of Socioeconomic Position and Working Conditions," *Obesity Research,* 13 (2005):2169–77.

6. D.L. Sherrill, K. Kotchou, S.F. Quan, "Association of Physical Activity and Human Sleep Disorders," *Archives of Internal Medicine,* 158, no. 17 (September 28, 1998):1894-98, http://archinte.ama-assn.org/cgi/reprint/158/17/1894.

7. M.L. Irwin, Y. Yasui, C.M. Ulrich, D. Bowen, R.E. Rudolph, R.S. Schwartz, M. Yukawa, E. Aiello, J.D. Potter, A. McTiernan, "Effect of Exercise on Total and Intra-abdominal Body Fat in Postmenopausal Women: A Randomized Controlled Trial," *JAMA*, 289, no. 3 (January 15, 2003):323–30, http://jama.ama-assn.org/cgi/content/full/289/3/323?ijkey=2ffd96d981677fb09007213e18cda542e6ed4cc0.

8. Qi Sun, Jing Ma, Hannia Campos, Susan Hankinson, JoAnn Manson, Meir Stampfer, Kathryn M. Rexrode, Walter Willett, Frank Hu, "A Prospective Study of Trans Fatty Acids in Erythrocytes and Risk of Coronary Heart Disease," *Circulation,* 115 (April 10, 2007):1858–65.

9. Ann Hettinger, "Rest Assured," Prevention, 59, no. 12 (December 2007):48.

10. Ann Hettinger, "Rest Assured," Prevention, 59, no. 12 (December 2007):48.

Chapter 4

1. Lawrence Rudel, Janice D. Wagner, John Jeffrey Carr, Kate Jones, Janet Sawyer, and Kathryn Kelly, "Trans Fat Leads to Weight Gain Even on Same Total Calories, Animal Study Shows," presented at the 66th annual Scientific Sessions of the American Diabetes Association in Washington, D.C., 2006.

2. Philip S. Chua, "Air Travel: Medical Tips," Heart to Heart Talk, CEBU Cardiovascular Center, (2003), http://www.cebudoctorsuniversity.edu/hospital/cardio/chua2.html.

3. J.W. Pennebaker, J.K. Kiecolt-Glaser, and R. Glaser, "Disclosure of Traumas and Immune Function: Health Implications for Psychotherapy," Journal of Consulting and Clinical Psychology, 56 (1988):239–45.

Chapter 5

1. Penny M. Kris-Etherton, Thomas A. Pearson, Ying Wan, Rebecca L. Hargrove, Kristin Moriarty, Valerie Fishell, and Terry D Etherton, "High Monounsaturated Fatty Acid Diets Lower Both Plasma Cholesterol and Triacylglycerol Concentrations," American Journal of Clinical Nutrition, 70 (1999):1009–15.

2. "Good Fats, Bad Fats—What You Need to Know," Health-e Woman, 1, no. 24 (June 6, 2007), http://www.ebsconewsletter.com/sunhealthwomen/e_article000832202.cfm?x=b11,0,w

Chapter 6

1. Steven Reinberg, "Excess Pounds Raise Women's Cancer Risk," HealthDay (November 7, 2007), http://body.aol.com/condition-center/breast-cancer/news/article/_a/excess-pounds-raise-womens-cancer-risk/n20071107090309990041.

Chapter 9

1. S.K. Park, J.H. Park, Y.C. Kwon, H.S. Kim, M.S. Yoon, and H.T. Park, "The Effect of Combined Aerobic and Resistance Exercise Training on Abdominal Fat in Obese Middle-Aged Women," Journal of Physiological Anthropology and Applied Human Science, 22, no. 3 (May 2003):129–35.

2. K. Tanaka, D.J. Lee, Y. Nakata, T. Okura, K. Ohkawara, "Effects of Aerobic Exercise and Obesity Phenotype on Abdominal Fat Reduction in Response to Weight Loss," International Journal of Obesity, 29, no. 10 (2005):1259–66.

3. I. Giannopoulou, L.L. Ploutz-Snyder, R. Carhart, R.S. Weinstock, B. Fernhall, S. Goulopoulou, and J.A. Kanaley, "Exercise Is Required for Visceral Fat Loss in Postmenopausal Women with Type 2 Diabetes," *Journal of Clinical Endocrinology & Metabolism,* 90, no. 3 (2005):1511–18.

4. Melinda L. Irwin, Yutaka Yasui, Cornelia M. Ulrich, Deborah Bowen, Rebecca E. Rudolph, Robert S. Schwartz, Michi Yukawa, Erin Aiello, John D. Potter, and Anne McTiernan, "Effect of Exercise on Total and Intra-abdominal Body Fat in Postmenopausal Women," *JAMA,* 289 (2003):323–30.

5. "Depression and Anxiety: Exercise Eases Symptoms," *MayoClinic.com* (October 23, 2006), http://www.mayoclinic.com/health/depression-and-exercise/MH00043.

6. Michele Stanten, Prevention's Firm Up in 3 Weeks: Trim and Tone Your Trouble Zones for Your *Best Body Ever* (Emmaus, PA: Rodale Inc., 2004): 9–10.

7. K. Clarke, J. Freeland-Graves, D. Klohe-Lehman, T. Milani, H. Nuss, and S. Laffrey, "Promotion of Physical Activity in Low-Income Mothers Using Pedometers" *Journal of the American Dietetic Association,* 107 (2007):962–67.

8. Rafael F. Escamilla, Clare Lewis, Duncan Bell, Gwen Bramblet, Jason Daffron, Steve Lambert, Amanda Pecson, Rodney Imamura, and Alan Hreljac, "An Electromyographic Analysis of Plank and Swiss Ball Exercises: Training and Rehabilitation Implications," *Medicine & Science in Sports & Exercise,* 39, no. 5 (May 2007): S259.

9. http://www.fhcrc.org/about/pubs/center_news/2004/apr15/sart3.html

10. Anne J. Blood and Robert J. Zatorre, "Intensely Pleasurable Responses to Music Correlate with Activity in Brain Regions Implicated in Reward and Emotion," *Proceedings of the National Academy of Sciences,* 98, no. 20 (September 25, 2001):11818–23.

11. Charles F. Emery, Evana T. Hsiao, Scott M. Hill, and David J. Frid, "Short-Term Effects of Exercise and Music on Cognitive Performance among Participants in a Cardiac Rehabilitation Program," *Heart & Lung: The Journal of Acute and Critical Care,* 32, issue 6 (November/December 2003): 368–73.

Chapter 10

1. "With Obesity on the Rise, Dieting a Constant Concern," *Calorie Control,* 29 (Fall 2007), http://www.caloriecontrol.org/pdf/ccc%20comm%20fall07_3.pdf.

2. Willard Bishop, "Making Healthy Eating Easier," *Shopping for Health 2006,* survey by *Prevention* magazine (2006).

3. Bruce Goldfarb, "TV Plays Role in Compulsive Snacking," *DOC News,* 4, no. 8 (August 1, 2007), http://docnews.diabetesjournals.org/cgi/content/full/4/8/12-a.

Index

Underscored page references indicate boxed text and tables.
Boldface references indicate photographs.

Flat Belly Diet!

ONLINE

Here's just a sampling of what you'll get by signing up for the Flat Belly Diet online subscription service at **flatbellydiet.com**:

■ **Daily Video Inspiration and Tips** from *Flat Belly Diet* coauthors Liz Vaccariello and Cynthia Sass, MPH, RD

■ **Easy-to-Manage Food Logs and Meal Plans** that can be customized to your calorie needs

■ **Extensive Community** so you can connect with other Flat Belly Dieters, read success stories, recruit buddies, journal, and stay motivated

■ **Access to Expert Help** to answer your questions and help you meet your goals

SIGN UP TODAY FOR YOUR 10-DAY RISK-FREE TRIAL AT:

flatbellydiet.com/bookoffer

FIRM UP FAST WITH
PREVENTION FITNESS DVDs.

200936501

No matter what your goal, from building better cardiovascular health to shedding excess pounds, odds are Prevention Fitness Systems has an easy-to-follow DVD to help you achieve it. And since each has been designed by the fitness editors of *Prevention* magazine, you know that they're safe, effective, and made with your total health in mind.

AVAILABLE IN STORES NOW!
www.prevention.com/shop